MEMO

OF T...

IODINE SURGEON

John Lionel Stretton

J.P., M.R.C.S., L.R.C.P.(Lond.), L.S.A.(Eng.)

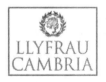

LLYFRAU
CAMBRIA

First published in the United Kingdom in 2012 by
Cambria Books; Carmarthenshire, Wales, United Kingdom

DEDICATION

Unusually, I dedicate this book to its author, and my great-grandfather, the late John Lionel Stretton.

For over seventy years Lionel's manuscript has lain in the family archives, awaiting publication. Now that this moment is finally realised, there can be only one person, John Lionel Stretton, to whom I, as the agent of this publication, can dedicate his book.

Chris Stretton, Lionel's great grandson and editor

FOREWORD

John Lionel Stretton, born on 20th September 1860, is my late great-grandfather.

Lionel was the third generation of surgeons in the family. Following his grandfather, William Birch of Barton-under-Needwood, he started his medical career as apprentice to his father, Samuel, in 1877, before becoming a celebrated surgeon in his own right. In his long career at Kidderminster hospital he performed over 40,000 operations and was responsible for many improvements to the hospital and the services that it provided to the community.

In addition to his unstinting service to the local population, Lionel left a legacy for which the whole world can be grateful. He was responsible for the introduction of tincture of iodine to sterilise the skin, several surgical inventions and development of a range of aseptic hospital equipment.

When he retired in 1938, in response to encouragement from his many friends and colleagues, Lionel put pen to paper, producing a book for the general reader entitled "Fifty-six Years a Surgeon - Recollections and Reflections". Trying to get this published in 1940, he received only rejections and must have been bitterly disappointed that he never saw it on the bookshelves before his death in 1943.

Thankfully, a copy of the manuscript survived and, finally, I am now able to publish it. In the process of bringing the original, typewritten manuscript to print I was curious to find out more about the man, not least to take this opportunity to fully recognise and publicise his innovative and pioneering contributions to medicine.

Lionel's style of writing is still fresh today thus I have been able to leave the original manuscript unchanged, although it must be admitted that one or two of the chapters are not as stimulating as others. On the other hand, I have added photographs and Addenda to incorporate material that tells more of Lionel's story, particularly Addendum 1, which reprints papers and letters concerning the introduction of iodine, and Addendum 7, which contains copies of two newspaper articles about him and his obituary from the British Medical Journal.

Being written as a collection of experiences from his working life *by* Lionel, rather than *about* him, this inevitably leaves us with questions about aspects of his life that he has not described. By coincidence another book, published concurrently with this one, fills in many of the gaps. If you are interested to know more about Lionel's life, and the family's three generations of service to the Kidderminster hospital and the local community, I would encourage you to read 'Dr Stretton, I presume', by Kidderminster local historian Nigel Gilbert.

Lionel was patently a 'local character' and much of his persona seeps from the following pages. As an example, he was rarely without his top-hat and recalls:

> "This loyalty to my top hat has led to some amusing incidents. In the early days of my practice one of my brothers dared me to ride wearing my top hat and frock-coat through the town and up the hill to the hospital on a high bicycle, the so-called penny-farthing. I did it, and a most ridiculous object I must have appeared!"

His story tells of very different times, records his strong views on a wide range of topics and is a fascinating and entertaining read.

Chris Stretton, editor
Llandysul, Carmarthenshire, Wales
2012

ACKNOWLEDGEMENTS

First, and foremost, I would like to thank my great-grandfather for writing the original manuscript, without which this book would not exist. Then there are those who have kept it safe in the years since Lionel completed his work: these include my father, Lionel James Stretton and my brother Jeremy Stretton.

In addition to the manuscript itself, the family archive of documents and photographs has proven to be a significant resource for this project. I am indebted to my late uncle, Antony John Stretton, for collating and retaining all this material over the years.

In my initial attempts to publish the book I approached many of the traditional publishers but, just as Lionel had experienced over seventy years ago, none were very helpful. Chris Jones, of Cambria Books, came as a breath of fresh air and I am most grateful to him for his help in publishing the book without me having to mortgage the house!

To supplement the original text, I have included photographs and contemporary published material from a number of sources and I am most grateful to the following organisations for their help in researching items and permissions to reproduce the material:

The British Medical Journal

Express Newspapers

Kidderminster Library

Kidderminster Medical Society and members

Kidderminster NHS Trust Centre – Education Centre

Kidderminster Shuttle

The Lancet

The Royal College of Nursing

Not being a 'Kidderminster Local', I have been helped in compiling the book by local historian, Nigel Gilbert, and am most appreciative of his assistance in this respect.

I am also indebted to Angela Bailey Haycock, Education Centre Manager at the Kidderminster NHS Treatment Centre at the time of research, since retired, for providing a number of the historic photographs that I have been able to include in the book.

My thanks are also due to members of the Kidderminster Medical Society, particularly, Barrie Davies, Dr Paul Newrick, John Murray and Timothy Wadsworth.

To complete the project, and present the book in a worthy cover, I was lucky to meet Nicola Clare Symberlist in a local business meeting. I'm sure you will agree that the cover design is first class and I am especially grateful to Nicola for her excellent work in producing a cover that admirably reflects the book's contents and Lionel's 'iodine' association.

Finally, my thanks are due to my wife, Sarah, for completing the job of checking and proof-reading the whole book before committing to print.

PREFACE

Many of my friends and colleagues have repeatedly urged me to write a book. Having known something of my work, listened to some of the many addresses I have given, and read some of the papers I have written, they appear to think that my experiences may be of interest to the general public. Whether their opinion is well founded remains to be seen.

I wish to place on record here my sincere thanks for the invaluable services rendered to me by my friend and secretary, Miss Susan Smith; but for her unfailing help and encouragement this book would never have been completed.

I have no wonderful tales of adventure to tell, no hairbreadth escapes by land or sea or in the air, no personal experience of famine, pestilence, or actual warfare, to relate. Most of my life has been spent in the provincial town of Kidderminster, an industrial centre that has grown up amidst some of the most beautiful scenery of the whole country. I do not flatter myself that I can teach humanity how to avoid trouble, nor can I disclose an infallible scheme for making this world a better and a happier place. But a man who has lived for nearly eighty years and spent nearly sixty years in active work as a doctor, in general and surgical practice, and on the staff of a hospital, can hardly fail to have garnered some useful experience, to have passed through thrilling incidents, and to have acquired definite views on life, its humours, its problems, and its lessons. Some of these experiences and views I have described on different occasions when giving addresses or reading papers, some of which will appropriately find a place in this book.

I resigned from the active honorary staff of the hospital at the end of 1938, when on the invitation of the Committee I accepted the position of Honorary Consulting Surgeon. I still act as a consulting surgeon in private practice and I hold various offices: Justice of the Peace of the Borough of Kidderminster; Chairman of the Local Emergency Committee of the Worcester and Bromsgrove Area; Chairman of the County of Worcester Local Medical and Panel Committee - an office I have held continuously since the establishment of the National Health

Insurance Scheme in 1912; and President of the Kidderminster Medical Society, which position I have held for more than thirty years.

All these offices entail a certain amount of more or less regular work, since I accept no position whose duties I am not prepared to carry out. But they do not absorb all my time and energies; hence my decision to comply with the suggestions of my friends and complete the preparation of this book, the materials for which I have been gradually accumulating for the past twenty years.

John Lionel Stretton
Kidderminster
1940

This Preface, by John Lionel Stretton, was Chapter 1 in his original manuscript

CONTENTS

CHAPTER I

EARLY YEARS AND RECOLLECTIONS

Birth. Grandparents. My father. Proneness to accidents. Earliest recollections.
Earthquakes. First operation. A dog-bite and its sequel. The brain in early life.

I was the third son in a family of twelve boys and three girls and was
born on the 20th September, 1860, at Kidderminster, where my father,
Samuel Stretton, had a large general practice extending beyond the town
into the surrounding country districts. He was the fourth son of William
Weston Stretton, of Leicester, a man of character and strong views.
When I went to stay with him as a child he lived on the outskirts of
Leicester.

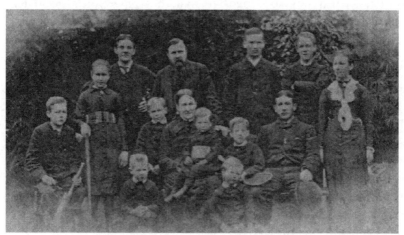

Samuel and Kate Stretton with their family circa 1880
John Lionel is back, left

I never heard of his doing any work, but he was a Justice of the Peace
and he used to go down to the town every morning and often sat on the

13

Bench. He impressed upon me the importance of the homely virtues of neatness, punctuality, and the regular payment of accounts. One Wednesday morning I was walking with him on his way to the Bench. We called at his tailor's to ask if his new suit was finished. The tailor said, "No, Mr. Stretton, I am afraid we have not finished the suit, but you shall have it on Saturday." The old gentleman told him he was not to think of sending a new suit to him on a Saturday. He said he had ordered it to wear to church; he was not going to church in anybody else's clothes, and he would certainly not pay for them until he had tried them on. At the very latest they must be sent to him on Friday, to give him time to try them on. If they were satisfactory he could pay for them on Saturday and go to church in his own clothes on Sunday. Whether this was meant as a lesson to me I do not know, but he there and then read me a homily on the desirability of always paying for anything when you had it and never ordering anything unless you had the money to pay for it. I hope I have profited by that advice.

He was fond of hunting, lived in ease and comfort, and kept a good table, though there was no extravagance. When I stayed with him a pudding was always served before the meat, which was the custom in those days. Meat was so expensive that they gave you a good feed of pudding first in the hope that you would not want so much meat afterwards.

My grandfather was a great judge of port wine and kept the very finest vintages. He considered that when a bottle was opened it ought to be finished and not kept for another day. He used to dine at 2 o'clock, and he would sit all the afternoon and drink at the wine till the bottle was finished. I never saw him in the slightest degree the worse for drink; he drank port wine, but nothing else at the same time or immediately afterwards. He had no sympathy with anybody who could not eat this, that, or the other. I have known him eat sausage, followed by toasted cheese and mushrooms for supper at 9 o'clock and go to bed at 10, feeling no ill effects afterwards.

When I ventured to suggest to him that that kind of diet would not agree with me he would pat his stomach and say, "Nonsense! I just put them down there and tell them to be good." He lived into his ninety-second year and died of old age. His wife, a very charming old lady, lived

14

to be seventy-eight. I was present when they celebrated their golden wedding. The family gave them a gold tea service, which has been handed down as an heirloom and is now in the possession of his great-grandson. This was the first of three golden wedding celebrations in my family; the second was that of my parents, the third was my own.

My mother was the third daughter of William Birch, of Barton-under-Needwood. Birch of Barton was a very remarkable man. He was lecturer on midwifery at St. Bartholomew's Hospital, London, but he had to go and live in the country for reasons of health. He settled in Barton and, in addition to his general practice there, he established a large consulting practice, which extended all over the Midlands. He will be referred to again later in connection with a letter to me from Luther Holden.

Some curious stories are related about Birch of Barton. He used to attend an old lady who always gave him two guineas: two golden sovereigns and two shillings. As was the custom in those days, the fee was wrapped up in silver paper and put into the hand of the physician as he went away. On one occasion the old lady gave him his fee as usual, wrapped up in silver paper, and he put it in his pocket and went off. When he had gone about a mile on his way home he opened the silver paper and found that the old lady had given him four gelatine lozenges instead of the two guineas. He stopped the coachman, drove back, and explained to his patient that she had made a mistake, whereupon, with many apologies, she rectified it.

On another occasion Birch went in consultation to see the wife of a nobleman. After a long interview in which the two doctors gave their directions to her husband they drove away. When they had reached about halfway up the long avenue that formed the drive they heard a noise of shouting behind them. A footman came up and said his lordship was very sorry, but he had forgotten whether her ladyship was to have rice pudding or sago. Birch turned to the footmen and said, "Tell his lordship that she is to have rice pudding and on no account sago." They then drove on, and the doctor who had called him in consultation said, "Mr. Birch, will you kindly tell me what there is in sago pudding that the old lady must not have." "I don't know," said Birch, "but they asked if she was to have rice or sago, and if I had said it did not matter they would have thought nothing of us."

Mr. Birch had a large family and died when he was about sixty-eight; his wife lived to be about seventy-eight. My own father and mother lived to be respectively eighty-eight and seventy-six. Hence I come of a long-lived family on both sides, and of families in which there were early marriages and many children. I used to go and stay with both my paternal and maternal grandparents and had the advantage of a great deal of instruction from them. They always set before me high ideals, which I have tried to keep undimmed.

My father had been in the Crimea, as a civil surgeon, with Spencer Wells, Rolleston, Budd, and others; he returned in 1856, at the end of the war. He had wanted to go into a dragoon regiment, but at a family conference on the subject it was decided that unless one of his wealthy old aunts would give him £300 a year he must refuse the commission that had been offered him. The £300 a year was not forthcoming. The man who got the commission instead of him was killed in his first engagement. It does not, of course, follow that my father would have been killed, because he might not have been just in the same place.

This reminds me, however, of an interesting observation I have made. Some families are much more prone than others to lose some of their members in war. Why should this be? Is the instinct of self- preservation greater in some families than in others? It is not because they are cowards and skulk behind. We all know that in the Great War a good many families lost three or four boys, killed perhaps directly they got out to the front. One of my brothers had three sons fighting. Two of them were at that awful landing at Gallipoli and afterwards in some of the worst of the fighting in France. These boys fought through the whole of the war and were never even wounded. One of them told me he went out with a platoon of thirty; only two of them came back, of whom he was one. Another told me that his pal, who was standing next to him, was blown to pieces by a shell, while he himself remained entirely unhurt.

A similar curious fact can be observed with regard to accidents, both in families and in individuals. It is well known in the medical world that some people are singularly prone to accidents. They have a series of them and break numerous bones on different occasions; others go through life without ever suffering the slightest mishap.

16

My father began his medical career as an apprentice to his uncle, a doctor in Leicester. He afterwards went to St. Bartholomew's and eventually became a House Surgeon there. He bought his Kidderminster practice in 1856 and married in the following year. He had only a few days' honeymoon and brought his bride back to a house in Church Street - at that time the Harley Street of Kidderminster - where he lived for twelve months. The first night after his return from his honeymoon he was called up to a patient. Twenty-five years later I returned from my honeymoon to the very same house, and the night after my return I was called up to the wife of the patient to whom my father had been called up the night after he returned from his honeymoon. Unlike my father, who had a strange desire to be always changing his place of abode, I lived in that house for fifty-six years, leaving it only in 1938.

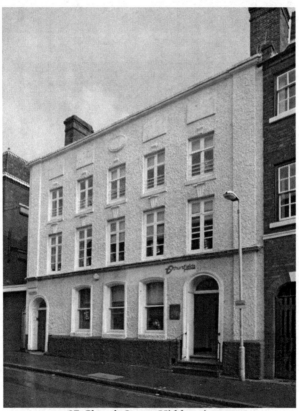

27 Church Street, Kidderminster
Picture taken 2012

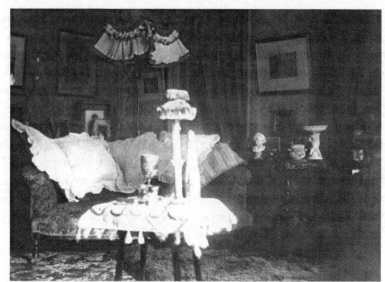

27 Church Street – Drawing Room

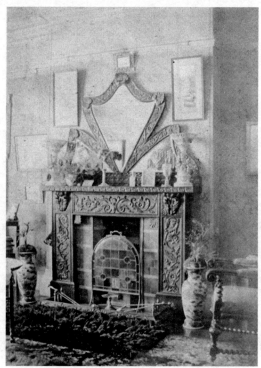

27 Church Street – Dining Room

18

As already stated, I was born in 1860. I had a wonderful old nurse and I cannot help thinking I can remember being handed to her when I was a month old. My mother and others often said that I imagined my early recollections, but I think I convinced them that it was not all imagination when I described the rides I used to enjoy in a pannier on a pony. This pony was disposed of before I was eighteen months old.

I remember perfectly a rather serious earthquake shock that happened in the night, when I was less than four years old. It woke me up and my old nurse put her head out of the window, shouting out to inquire what the matter was. Most people in the street were at their windows. It sounded to me as if something big had come up against the house, which seemed to shiver and shake, and there was a horrible rumbling noise. Some forty years later there was another earthquake shock in the night. It woke me up and I knew in a moment what it was, because I remembered the earlier one so well and it was exactly the same kind of thing.

I distinctly remember being taken by my nurse on a visit to London when I was still in frocks and probably about three or four years old. She took me to the zoo, where I saw the lions fed. I remember also her taking me to see one of her brothers, who was an optician in Beak Street. In after years, when I was a student at St. Bartholomew's, I used to go to that selfsame brother's to dinner, and I remembered the stairs and everything as being just the same. That nurse was a good old soul and she was devoted to us during the ten or twelve years she was with us. When I was a medical student in London it was one of my pleasures to go to tea with her occasionally on Sundays at Brixton, where she lived with a niece between the time of her retirement from service and her death.

While I was still a child I had made up my mind that I should be a surgeon. My mother often put before me the disadvantages of a surgeon's life, but it was of no avail. I was determined to follow my inclination. I used to drive with my father on his rounds and later I often rode on a pony beside him. I took every opportunity of visiting the hospital - then called the infirmary - and before I was ten years old I often went into the wards. I also got into our own dispensary whenever I could and saw various dressings and extractions of teeth. The first effort I made myself was when I was eleven years old. A wheelwright carried on his trade near our house and my brothers and I were constantly in his yard. I fear we must often have delayed and annoyed him, but he was very good-natured and never complained to our father about us.

One day he said to me, "Well, young sawbones, do you think you could pull out a tooth for me?" Even then I was cautious enough to ask him to open his mouth so that I could examine the tooth. It was a right upper molar just beginning to loosen. I agreed to undertake the operation. I rushed home and secured an old pair of forceps that my father had relegated to the tool-basket, and armed with these I returned. The old man sat on a log in his yard and I extracted the tooth. I rather fancy I failed to obtain any fee, but that did not interest me in those days. When my father found out about this he related the story to many of his friends, with the result that I had several extractions to perform, for which I received gratuities. My most important patient was my father himself. He afterwards explained that he allowed me to operate because he knew I should stop if he ordered me to do so. Should I? I remember he groaned, but I pulled out the tooth.

My mother was a wonderful woman. She had fifteen children and reared twelve of them. She was always at work for us and made all our clothes: she made my first knickerbockers out of my father's old clothes. It was to help her a little by keeping us out of her way that my father used to take us out with him on his rounds. There were certain of his patients' houses that we very much preferred to others, because the people who lived in them were in the habit of sending us out refreshments.

At one particular house the parlour-maid regularly brought us out glasses of milk, mince-pies, grapes, peaches, etc. There was always something for us children, and bread and cheese and beer for the coachman. That impressed me at the time and there was an interesting sequel. Some years later that parlour-maid married the gardener and they took on a small farm. Between thirty and forty years afterwards she had the misfortune to have her hand bitten by a dog. She went to a chemist and he rubbed some caustic on the wound in her hand, which healed up.

20

Six or eight months later she had a great deal of trouble in her house owing to the illness of some of her grandchildren. It upset her very much and lowered her vitality, with the result that her hand became red and swollen. The mischief increased. I had to make incisions in the palm and the dorsum of her hand; in spite of this the poison crept up her forearm necessitating further incisions. It then got into her upper arm and the limb became gangrenous. I recognised that the only way to save her life was to amputate her arm. She repeatedly refused to allow this. Her husband could not persuade her to it and he would not allow it to be done without her consent. I was determined that she should not die and I sat by her bedside for nearly two hours trying every possible means to persuade her to have the gangrenous arm removed, and at last I succeeded.

I performed the operation as soon as I could get the preparations made, and it saved her life. She lived for many years afterwards. About a week after the operation, when she was getting better, she said to me, "Ah, Sir, I know you have saved my life, but I should never have agreed to the operation only I suddenly thought of you sitting in your father's carriage when I used to bring you out milk and mince pies."

This case is interesting from another point of view. An action was brought against the owner of the dog that bit the old lady. I gave evidence at the trial and stated that in my opinion the condition was caused by germs that had remained latent in her system until her bodily vitality was so lowered that they were able to get the upper hand. This was a point that at that period had not been advanced, but the possibility is now a generally accepted fact. The judge accepted my opinion and awarded compensation.

In connection with my own early recollections, I have often in later life pondered on the brain. When does it first begin to function? I doubt if the period is constant. It probably differs in different individuals, as does also the development of other organs. It would be interesting to know the earliest time at which it has given proof of its reasoning capacity. Are the movements in utero voluntary? They are certainly performed by voluntary muscles. Some regard them as involuntary, but on many occasions I have felt blows from the babies in response to prods I have given to them from without. This is often called reflex action. But can reflex action take place unless the brain is functioning?

Apart from this, when does the brain begin really to understand? When does it begin to store knowledge? I have questioned many people. The majority of them cannot remember anything that happened during their first three or four years of life. I have never met anyone who professed to remember being born or any incident of his residence in utero.

I should expect a brain to begin storing knowledge before it is capable of reasoning, that is, drawing deductions from observations made. I can give a remarkable instance of this in a child ten months old. My daughter walked by herself when she was ten months old. At this age she once evaded her nurse and went into my bedroom. While she was there the door blew to and she was shut in. I think most children would have howled, but she did not. Instead of that she pushed a chair across the room to a bell-pull that hung from the ceiling. She mounted on that chair and pulled the bell for the servant, who went and liberated her. No doubt the child had noticed her mother ringing for the maid. She had stored that information in her brain and she possessed the reasoning power to apply it to secure her rescue from the room in which she was imprisoned.

Is there any record of an earlier exhibition of this function? Is there any proof that it cannot occur before birth? We cannot say, nor can we say with any certainty at what period of life the brain power begins to fail. It has been stated that at a certain age the brain cells are used up and that we are then incapable of absorbing new knowledge or of performing constructive work. This is not correct. The assertion may be true in some cases, but it is impossible to state any age at which it is applicable to all.

The custom in some occupations of insisting upon resignation at the age of sixty or sixty-five may be advantageous in the majority of instances, but it will deprive the community of a number of men who are capable of valuable work and whose experience can ill be spared.

As already indicated, the same variations are to be observed in early life. Some children show advanced knowledge and reasoning power at an earlier period than the average child. In these days of education such a precocious child may be unduly pushed forward, to its own detriment.

CHAPTER II

EDUCATION

Early teaching. Lying fallow. Boarding-school. King Charles I School, Kidderminster. Games. Coaching for preliminary professional examination. Speeches at school functions. Teaching of physiology. Heredity and environment. School sports. Per laborem ad honorem. Secrets of longevity. Tragedies of single child and childless marriage. Nature's laws. Science versus wealth. Choice of occupation. The "good old days."

Our early education was chiefly what we picked up rather than any formal instruction. We had various governesses, but I doubt whether they ever taught me very much. I remember doing a great many copies in copy-books. I know on one occasion when my mother was giving us a dictation I got into great trouble for spelling Europe Yourup. I still think it was a good way of spelling it. Spelling has never been a strong point with me, but in later life I have sometimes managed to conceal uncertainty of spelling by doubtful writing. I fancy that in my early years my brain lay fallow so far as lessons were concerned. That reminds me that a distinguished educationist once told me that he preferred to deal with boys whose brains had lain fallow until they were ten years of age. My own experience tends to support his view.

I went to a boarding-school when I was nine years old, but I was never well there and had to spend most of my time in the sick-room. Consequently, I was brought home to attend the King Charles I School, Kidderminster, usually called the Grammar School. I was then ten years old. I had a distaste for lessons and had always evaded them by every means I could think of, so I naturally found myself much behind my fellow-pupils of the same age.

My knowledge of arithmetic was confined to the fact that I had seen rows of figures put on a blackboard, a line drawn under them, and another row of figures put underneath the line. I had no idea that 1 + 2 made 3; subtraction and the multiplication tables were as sealed books to me. On my first morning at the Grammar School I was given a column of figures to add up. I looked at them for a short time, then made a row of figures underneath the line and thought sums were easy. I was complimented upon being so quick, but was much discomfited to find that I was quite wrong. However, a little kind and friendly explanation soon set me right and before I left school that morning I was able to add up a fair sum. I felt I had learnt more that day than in all my life before, but my heart fainted at my ignorance and I thought I should never learn all the other boys knew. Yet within a week I was working quite comfortably at fractions and I soon became an expert mathematician; I never found the slightest difficulty with Euclid and algebra. The probability is that the early lying fallow of my brain was of very great benefit to me later.

I never did any work that I could avoid at school. I spent all my available time in the playground and had sufficient brains to be able to hold my own in school by learning my lessons on the way home, so I managed to escape punishment. Classics I abhorred; mathematics I revelled in. I always felt a grievance against the Head Master. I protested to him against being asked to commit poetry to memory. I did not care whether the way was long and the wind was cold; it mattered nothing to me. I told the Head Master that I was quite willing to do double the amount of mathematics, natural philosophy, or anything of that kind, but I did not want to waste my time in learning poetry. He would not listen. I maintain that one of the great faults of education is this kind of cast-iron system with its rules applied to all alike. For a master to refuse to listen to a boy who has sufficient intelligence and initiative to make such a reasonable request seems to me inexcusable.

It was at games that I excelled. I was captain of the cricket and football teams and the leading spirit in some exciting paper-chases. I also won several prizes for running. At that time W.G. George was at the height of his fame and I ran against him several times.

While I was at school our family was regularly increasing. During one of the holidays my father sent the three eldest boys to Walsall to see the great W.G. Grace play in a cricket match, and very thoroughly we enjoyed it. On our return home we found that we had another brother. I do not suppose we realised that that was the reason we had been sent off out of the way, but it was.

I left school in 1876, not having passed any qualifying examination. I was then sent to a coach in Birmingham to be prepared for the preliminary examination of the Royal College of Surgeons, an examination that has since been given up. My coach was a classical scholar, a member of the medical profession, and a kind of recluse. He prided himself on the fact that no woman had been into his study for fifteen years. I went there every day by train and used to take books with me, which I studied on the journey there and back. I had only a short time for preparation, but I passed the examination in March, 1877. In April, 1877, I was apprenticed to my father, and this was the beginning of my professional training.

I have always taken an active interest in my old school, which I attended for six years. I was appointed one of the Governors of the School in 1925, and I still hold that office. I was President of the Old Carolians' Association from 1924 to 1932, and I have made many speeches on Prize Days, at the Old Carolians' Annual Dinner, and at other school functions. These speeches are on much the same lines as those made at other schools on similar occasions, but I will quote certain passages here because they illustrate my own views on education and kindred subjects.

> "Some of you will agree that there is one aspect of the question of education on which I am entitled to speak - the medical aspect. We hear nowadays (1901) a great deal about physical deterioration, the falling birth-rate, and the high rate of infant mortality. We know that quackery is rampant in the land and that last year the country spent £4,000,000 on quack medicines. All these facts indicate a great want of knowledge on the part of the public. It is of paramount importance that all boys should have some training in elementary physiology and the personal care of health. I know many instances of boys who have irretrievably ruined their health

27

simply and solely through ignorance. Our bodies are given to us as a sacred trust and it is our duty to take care of them, and to see that our children know how to take care of them. This is impossible unless they possess some knowledge of the structure and functions of the body. The time spent at school is a period of development and growth; it is a period pregnant with future manhood's fate. All these matters need to be looked at from the scientific point of view, and if this is beyond the scope of the schoolmaster it would be an advantage to associate with him a man who has had special training in the subject. I know I shall be told that the school curriculum is already overburdened. It seems to me that the time necessary for such an important subject should be made; moreover, I believe the time has come when the curriculum should be cast into the melting-pot and some subjects be eliminated or considerably curtailed? "

"I feel it is impossible to put education upon a scientific basis until we have cleared the ground and come to some understanding as to which is the more important factor in forming the character of the growing race — heredity or environment. No doubt all people admit that both are important, but there are differences of opinion as to which takes precedence. I was brought up in the old belief that you cannot make a silk purse out of a sow's ear. I am certain that no amount of education will transform into a good citizen a man who was born to become a criminal. You may say that education might at least improve him. It might do so, but on the other hand it might have an opposite effect. A rogue is bad enough, but a trained rogue is a greater danger to Society. If you admit that I have made out my case so far, you must also admit that one of the most important topics needing consideration in these days (1910) is that of Eugenics."

"Your Head Master reminds me that today is the anniversary of Waterloo. It has often been said that that battle was won on the playing-fields of Eton, and there is no doubt that the spirit engendered by sport at our public schools is of great value in warfare. Much as we hope that wars will cease I am afraid the time has not yet come (1924), and though I trust that you boys may not be called upon to bear arms I feel confident that if and when you are you will be guided by the principles you have learnt on the playing-fields here, that you will strive to win and will acquit yourselves as all true Britons should."

"But in your zeal for sport you must not forget the other and the more important side of your education. Your brain must work as well as your body. It is not only yourselves you have to consider, but your country. Each individual, no matter how humble his sphere, bears his own responsibility and can do his share in upholding the honour and greatness of his country. It rests with you to carry on the traditions of those noble men who have assisted to build up the great Empire to which we have the privilege to belong."

"The anniversary of Waterloo inevitably reminds us of Wellington and of the words of Tennyson: 'The path of duty was the way to glory.' The same idea is briefly expressed in your school motto - Per laborem ad honorem - and I would urge you to take this to heart and act upon it. The service of your country and of your fellow-men will give you more happiness than can be obtained from the pursuit of any selfish pleasure, and when the time comes for you to depart hence you will have the satisfaction of knowing that you have not lived in vain."

"It is probable that there is a natural limit to human life and that this limit will never be increased. I cannot give you the figure, because it has not been agreed upon. I think it is more than the Psalmist's three score years and ten, but it does not reach one hundred."

"No doubt you would like to know now (1927) how you can ensure that you will live to this limit. In my own profession a considerable number of old men have disclosed the secrets of longevity for the benefit of the rising generation. These secrets afford very interesting reading. Unfortunately, they vary considerably; and when doctors differ, who shall decide? One of them tells us that the prime factor in attaining advanced years is to avoid all alcoholic drinks. Of course he is a teetotaller, and he

29

omits to mention the fact that many old men have taken alcohol regularly."

"Another writer tells us that exercise is the prime factor. Of course he is a golfer, and he omits to mention the fact that many old men have taken very little exercise. I remember a distinguished physician, who lived to be eighty-three, stating his opinion of the craze for exercise. He said, 'I walk only from the front door to my carriage, and I would not walk that if I could get someone to carry me.' Another advises you about your clothing and may advocate your discarding a hat. Some say a tall hat causes baldness. You have in front of you a standing refutation of this statement."

"It is quite evident that all the secrets of attaining old age cannot be correct, and therefore if I add to the list my own secret it will not create confusion. If you desire to live more than the average number of years there are two main factors to be taken into account: heredity and environment. You must arrange to be born of long-lived parents; you will then inherit not only the germ plasm but also the bumps of self-preservation and early marriage. You will avoid riotous companions and seek a healthy environment; you will live a life of physiological righteousness, which means moderation in all things, and you will not worry; remember that worry is to a large extent what we make for ourselves."

"This is not the place for me to deliver a lecture on birth control, but it is an opportunity for me to draw your attention to the luxurious living of the present day (1928), to remind you of the fall of the greatest Empire of bygone days, and to point to the tragedy of the single child and the even greater tragedy of the childless marriage. These are subjects upon which I feel very strongly. I hope you will ponder over these facts."

"School is a very important section of environment, but it cannot create a genius. It trains you and cultivates your intellect; but you will find in all schools that some boys win prizes, while others, with equal opportunities, will be unable to win them. It is the same in the professions, in business, and in sport. We are not all equal. This is one of Nature's laws, and it is one of the valuable lessons we learn at school."

"School teaches us how to work and also the advantages of work. One of the main objects of work is to earn your living. Some men find it difficult to earn enough money to live upon, whereas others earn vast fortunes. There are men of science who have made discoveries of enormous importance to their country; some of them have made inventions that have enabled other men to gain fortunes, while they themselves have had difficulty to live. Yet if you were to question these men of science you would find that they would not relinquish their work to take up a money-making occupation. It is probable that scientific men are happier than money-making men. There are many good things in this life that cannot be bought with money. Money cannot buy happiness or peace of mind; it cannot wipe out the memory of mean and sordid acts."

"When you leave school you have to choose your occupation. In making this choice do not be led astray by the lure of money. Choose an occupation that you can enjoy for its own sake, and, having chosen it, determine to excel at it. You will make mistakes. But do not be discouraged; you may learn more from a mistake than from a success."

"When I was a boy my grand-parents and my parents often talked to me about the good old days and what a much better world it was when they were young. I may have talked to my children about the good old days, but what surprises me most is to hear my children themselves speak of the good old days. It appears that one generation is enough to create this feeling."

"I can remember the time when I had to walk to Worcester. I have ridden there on horseback and have driven there in a carriage. I have ridden there on a wooden bicycle with iron tires, on a high bicycle, and on a safety bicycle. I now (1930) go by motor-car in less than half the time and in greater comfort. I have not yet travelled in an aero-plane, but I believe this method of travelling will be considerably developed and I imagine that the pedestrians of the future may have exciting times dodging the wreckage from collisions in the air."

"I have seen the coming of the telephone, the gramophone, and the wireless. In my own profession I have seen the work of Pasteur and Lister revolutionise surgery and enable us to achieve success such as was undreamt of when I started practice. Instruments of precision, electricity and the X-rays have given us advantages which it is difficult to estimate. As a consequence of these modern improvements the student of today is apt to belittle the work of his forbears. He has no justification for such an attitude."

"It has been my privilege to be intimately acquainted with some of the great men in my profession. They had only their own observation, judgement, and experience to rely upon, and I still marvel at the skill and clinical acumen that they attained in the absence of the aids that are at our disposal today. It is sad to think of the horrors of the operating-rooms in pre-anaesthetic days. The sufferings of the patients must have been appalling. If those were the good old days we may thank God that we did not live in them."

"I have lived happily under the conditions that have existed during my life - conditions, mark you, that were condemned by the previous generation. I advise you to think of the good present days, instead of the good old days, and I hope you will live happily under the conditions to which you will be subject during your lives. Inventions and discoveries will still cause changes in the world and alter the conditions that obtain today. But whatever changes may come, the laws of Nature and the laws of God will remain unchanged. Love, honour and truth will remain with us for ever and you must try to keep them constantly before you. If you are not the master of your fate you will surely strive to be the captain of your soul. You will have successes, you will have failures. You will meet with disappointments, you will be subject to temptations, and you will be obliged to make momentous decisions. In making these decisions think of your old School, think of your mother, and consult your conscience, which she taught you to consult. It will tell you what is right. Then take the path of rectitude, and you will find that it is the path to happiness."

CHAPTER III

PROFESSIONAL TRAINING

Apprentice to my father. System of apprenticeship. Dispensing. Unqualified assistant. St. Bartholomew's Hospital, London. First failure in examination. System of examination. Serious illness. M.R.C.S., L.S.A., L.R.C.P. Assistant Anaesthetist at St Bartholomew's. Deputy casualty physician. Resignation of appointments. Partnership with my father. Letters.

As already stated, I was apprenticed to my father, who had an extensive general practice, in 1877. In the light of all my later experience, and in spite of all that has been done to improve the education of medical men, I still consider that the old system of apprenticeship was the best. We have nothing to equal it nowadays. The present-day teachers and the powers that be consider themselves vastly superior to our ancestors, but I sometimes wonder whether the bygone generations were not wiser than we were, at any rate in certain respects. Even now, if I had my time to come over again, I should choose to be educated by the same system as was followed in my early medical training, when boys of sixteen or seventeen years of age were apprenticed to general practitioners.

I attended at our dispensary every morning at 9 o'clock. I learnt such practical points as the best methods of cleaning measures, washing, wrapping up and labelling bottles. I had to help the assistant to make up the medicines. I became familiar with all the various drugs, their appearance, their smell, and their taste - matters of no small importance. I learnt how to make mixtures, tinctures, infusions, pills, and plasters.

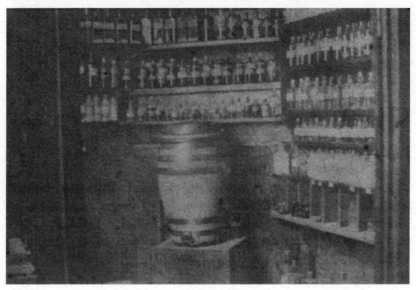
Dispensary

This is all scoffed at to-day, the result being that hardly one medical man in a thousand knows what medicines should look like, smell like, or taste like. More often than not the men nowadays prescribe various tablets and proprietary medicines. Owing to my early training and my practice since I believe I could still give the main constituents of most bottles of medicine that might be submitted for my inspection. I am not a great believer in medicines, but there is no doubt that some of them are of great value in the treatment of disease, and an elegant method of administering them is an asset that a general practitioner cannot afford to despise. Many men now think medicines should be made up by the chemist, a view from which I entirely dissent. I consider that every practitioner should make up his own medicines. I am quite willing to admit that doctors in the past have given their patients coloured or scented water and bread pills, and I maintain that they were perfectly justified in so doing.

If a patient has a prescription made up by different chemists he is apt to complain that the bottles of medicine are not exactly alike. Moreover, say what you like, the element of mystery is a very large factor in the treatment of disease and therefore it is far better that patients should not know what they are taking. I never let them know. If any patient says to me that the medicine is mostly water I always reply, "Yes, more than 80% of it is water; and how much water do you think there is in a strawberry?" They are astonished when I tell them it is more than 80%.

As an apprentice I learnt also the system of book-keeping, the prices of drugs, and the mysteries of fees. I used to go out with the assistant to see patients. I also visited the hospital and went round the wards with the house-surgeon.

Under the system of apprenticeship by the time a young man had finished his apprenticeship he was able to open abscesses, extract teeth, perform other minor operations, and use a thermometer and a stethoscope with more or less accuracy. He had an intimate acquaintance with all minor ailments and a more superficial one with serious complaints. He had also learnt how to deal with patients, using tact and discrimination.

In January, 1878, I went as unqualified assistant to a doctor who had a large general practice in and around a neighbouring town. I visited many patients with him and under his direction saw many patients in the dispensary and performed minor operations. After I had been with him for a few months he had an illness that confined him to bed for a fortnight, and I had to carry on the practice. One patient caused me much anxiety. I could not decide what was the matter with him, so I sent for my father to come and see him with me. To my great astonishment my father said to me as we entered the house: "Your patient is suffering from rheumatic fever." "How do you know that?" I asked. "I can smell him," was his reply, and he was right. That gave me a lesson that has been very useful to me many times since.

I resigned my assistantship in September 1878, and on the 1st October my father took me up to St. Bartholomew's Hospital. I was put to live in college and had a room on the ground floor, the most dismal room I had ever been in. I felt very miserable when I was left alone there with nothing to do. However, I soon found friends among my fellow-students, some of whom remained my fast friends as long as they lived. Looking back on this period I cannot help feeling how very important it is that one's early companions should be of the right sort. There were so many temptations in London and so many tragedies among the students of the hospital. I can quite conceive that I might have gone altogether wrong if I had been introduced into a fast set.

I was devoted to cricket and football and hitherto hard study had had little attraction for me. But in less than twenty-four hours at the hospital I learnt that if I was to succeed in my profession work - and very hard work - was necessary and that it would not do to let cricket and football distract my attention. I therefore packed up my football and cricket things and sent them home at once in order to remove temptation as far as possible. I felt almost overwhelmed with the task that was before me, especially when I compared myself with other students. There were probably over 700 of them in all, among whom were many university men. However, I set to work in earnest. I attended all the lectures, did a great deal of dissecting and kept regular hours for reading. The knowledge of chemistry, physiology, and anatomy that I had gained during my apprenticeship stood me in good stead when I entered the hospital, for I was able to learn them more easily than if I had been entirely a raw recruit. And when I went into the wards and the out-patient departments I was immediately placed at an enormous advantage, because I could do all the minor operations we were allowed to undertake with a degree of knowledge and skill never possessed by the students who had not been apprenticed, for the system of apprenticeship was even then becoming a thing of the past.

My reading was generally done between 6 and 10 at night, and after a little relaxation I went to bed at 11 p.m. Exercise was taken by walking; I had no bicycle. I was fortunate in possessing some relations in the West End, where I was often invited to dinner, especially on Sundays. My walks there and back gave me exercise and also some knowledge of London.

In 1880 I went up for the Royal College of Surgeons examination and failed. This seemed surprising, because at St. Bartholomew's I had been bracketed first in the physiology examination and I was second in the anatomy examination. The reason of my failure was that I had foolishly misread one of the questions. A very distinguished member of the profession wrote to my father about this, as follows:

"I was very much pained and surprised to find that your son had not passed the examination at the College of Surgeons and at once made some inquiries respecting the reason, but it was not necessary to inquire after I heard that, by a mistake of reading 'perineal' for 'pelvic' or vice\versa, he had answered one thing instead of another. I know that anyone who is unfortunate enough to make such a mistake cannot afterwards get through, however well he may do in the rest of the examination. But inasmuch as your son received the high honour that he did at our Anatomical Prize examination as well as that we considered him certain to pass among the very first from the whole school I think he need not be very miserable about it, but he must come up next time with good spirits and take care to be more careful in reading the questions, for the question he answered was much more difficult than the one he was asked but nevertheless counted as nothing in the marking."

This preliminary failure did not interfere with my career, but it was very annoying. I felt no grudge against the examiners; they could not have acted otherwise. It was the system of examination that was at fault, because it did not take into account the work that the men had done at their hospitals or schools. I maintain that in deciding all such questions the opinion of the teacher should be sought and should have very considerable weight.

In May, 1881, I contracted diphtheria and scarlet fever and was so ill that both my father[1] and my mother were sent for. In my five days of delirium I went to all sorts of places and did all sorts of peculiar things, which I remembered perfectly afterwards; but I want to put definitely on record that I never suffered in the very slightest degree; in fact, I had a jolly good time. That should be a great comfort to people who see their dear ones apparently in such terrible distress in similar circumstances. Of course I was intensely weak when I came round. I had to remain in the hospital for nearly two months, and all through the time of my convalescence I was treated with the utmost generosity. They gave me

---

[1] See Addendum 5.1

duck and green peas, asparagus and strawberries galore. Nothing was too good for me. Afterwards I had to be away in the country for two months.

In spite of the loss of these four months I went up for my final examination and on October 10th, 1881, I was a member of the Royal College of Surgeons, a few weeks after my twenty-first birthday. Soon afterwards I qualified as Licentiate of the Society of Apothecaries and Licentiate of the Royal College of Physicians. I was appointed Junior Assistant Anaesthetist at St. Bartholomew's and had a very pleasant time on the staff, though our hours of duty were long. I have given as many as fifty anaesthetics a day. I lived in the Hospital at this time and had many opportunities of acting as deputy for other men when they were out or away.

It is sometimes said that students see minor ailments among patients in the out-patient departments of hospitals. This is not correct. At St. Bartholomew's there was a sorting-out room where the casualty physicians and surgeons sorted out the cases without the presence of any students. On one occasion I acted as deputy casualty physician for six weeks. The duty largely consisted in sifting out the medical out-patients in the morning. I have seen as many as 250 of them in a couple of hours. We used to sit in a room with a door at each end. The patients were sent in by the porters at one door and went out at the other. I had in front of me tickets for all the different departments: ear, throat, ophthalmic, skin, and so on, and also out-patient and in-patient tickets. I also had a box of coloured cards, each colour representing some five or six different medicines. I had to sift the patients out. Obviously if a man had a rash I gave him a ticket for the skin department; if he had something wrong with an eye, a ticket for the ophthalmic department, and so on. It was quite easy to deal with this and also to see if a person was ill enough to be given an in-patient ticket. The difficulty was to cope with the medicines and the people who were not really very ill but wanted a dose of medicine. Some of them were brazen enough to come in and point to the ticket they wanted. I always remember the story of an old lady who lived in one of the streets in the neighbourhood and who was famed for her wonderful cough lozenges, of which she sold quantities. It was ultimately found out that the principal ingredient of these lozenges was the 'hospital linctus', for which she used to come regularly.

40

It was really wonderful that in spite of these somewhat haphazard methods of diagnosis hardly ever was a mistake made. The facial expression is one of the most valuable diagnostic signs. An observant and experienced medical man on walking through the wards of a hospital can tell you how the patients are, and what is the matter with a good many of them, even though he may never have seen them before. He can often tell what is the matter with people he may see in the streets.

All this experience in the Hospital was most valuable to me, and it was filling up the time until I could take on the other positions that I was to hold after the summer: that of House-Surgeon, and later that of Resident Midwifery Assistant.

Suddenly, early in August, 1882, I received a telegram summoning me home, because my father was very ill. I made all my arrangements and came home. The physician in attendance told me that unless I resigned my positions in London and came home to help my father he would not live long. He had a family of seven sons younger than myself to educate, so I had no choice. I immediately went back to London to hand in my resignations of the positions I had been looking forward to holding. I then wrote to my father that I was willing to give up my London career, which I felt to be pretty well assured, and come home to help him in any way I could. I left the terms to him and made only one condition that I must have a house to myself. In making that condition I showed wisdom beyond my years. After completing the arrangements for resigning my posts at St. Bartholomew's Hospital I left there on August 9th, 1882, and came to join my father in partnership.

In connection with my decision to resign my career in London I received a number of very gratifying letters, among them the two following.

Matthews Duncan wrote:

"I am sorry to lose your services which I anticipated having the advantage of. But you follow what you regard as the path of duty and that is right and proper also the path of happiness."

Luther Holden wrote:

"I send you the enclosed Testimonial with my best wishes for your happiness and success in our profession. And you will be happy and successful just in proportion to the amount of thought and good judgment which you show for your patients.

You begin your practice under most favourable auspices and under the best traditions. Your father is held in high esteem by all who know him and I know him well. Your grandfather - maternal - was looked up to as one of the best surgeons in England. Had he continued to live in London he was just the man to have led the town. Him also I knew well - and looked up to - as the type of a powerful surgeon, who had complete control over his patients. His will was supreme. His decision was courted by the highest and the lowest in the midland counties. He was the true King of men. He worked day and night. He drove the best blood horses – and exercised self-denial for the common good. He was beloved by most, feared by some, valued by all. BIRCH of BARTON is still a tradition.

Catch him playing cricket or lawn tennis or football! He knew that those with whom he played would not prize him professionally and he was right. Hard lines! But the true lines!"

CHAPTER IV

PARTNERSHIP AND EVENTS IN PRIVATE LIFE

Settlement in Kidderminster. Appointment on Hospital Staff. Medical Officer of workhouse. Marriage. Serious illness. Two golden weddings.

My father urged me to go away for a long holiday before actually beginning work as his partner. I preferred to get everything straight first, with the result that I never went for that holiday at all. I settled down in the house I was to live in for fifty-six years. I was able to furnish only two or three rooms completely and I did this out of money I had saved during my boyhood, chiefly gifts from rich uncles, grandfathers, godfathers, and others. My income was then very small. My sister came to keep house for me; we had an old man and his wife to look after the house and garden, and a boy acted as 'Buttons', answered the bell and valeted for me.

My father resigned from the hospital staff and I applied for the vacant position as honorary surgeon. In support of my application I had many testimonials from the leading physicians and surgeons at St. Bartholomew's Hospital, all of whom expressed their regret at my leaving there and their good wishes and confidence with regard to my future success in my professional career. Among the writers of these testimonials were: Norman Moore, James Paget, Luther Holden, W.S. Savory, Alfred Willett, W. Morrant Baker, Howard Marsh, James Shuter, W.J. Walsham, A.E. Cumberbatch, Henry T. Butlin, Dyce Duckworth, T. Lauder Brunton, J. Wickham Legg, J. Matthews Duncan, and Clement Godson. I had worked under and with these men and they were able to judge of my character and abilities.

I obtained the appointment at the hospital and resigned it only at the end of 1938. A later chapter will give more information about the hospital and my work there.

In 1882, as my father's partner, I was appointed Deputy Medical Officer of the Workhouse and District and Surgeon to the Kidderminster Lying-in Charity; the last-mentioned provided me with upwards of 100 midwifery cases a year.

My first two years at Kidderminster were very strenuous ones. I did practically all the work at the workhouse and in the parish district, and all our own dispensing and book-keeping. The practice increased to such an extent in these two years that I ultimately gave way to my father's advice that I should have an assistant.

I was married in April, 1884, having known my wife since childhood. In the year 1904, I had a serious illness which nearly cost me my life. After a heavy day's work I felt my arm itching in the evening and found there was a malignant pustule on the outer side of my left forearm. There had been a case of anthrax in the hospital and I might have got infected from it. This was before the days of anti-anthrax serum. Within half an hour of finding the pustule I had it excised under a general anaesthetic. I kept on with my work for several days, carrying my arm in a sling. My condition grew worse and when I found my temperature was 103°F, I went to bed. Within forty-eight hours I was delirious, with a temperature of over 105°F. I remained unconscious for five days. It is curious that the period of unconsciousness and the temperature were both similar to those I experienced in the illness of which I nearly died at St. Bartholomew's in 1881. On both occasions my life was despaired of. On this latter occasion eight members of the profession, including London consultants, said that I should die, but I did not. The delirium was different on this occasion, for I cannot remember a single thing from the time when I became unconscious until I woke up again. But I am quite clear that I did not suffer at all and, as previously indicated, it is very satisfactory to me to be able to comfort people by assuring them that delirious patients are not really suffering.

One of the physicians who saw me said that even if I did recover I should not be able to do any work for six months. In less than six weeks

I went into Nottinghamshire and performed an abdominal operation. The powers of recuperation are very great in some people. No doubt I lost a stone or two in weight, but as soon as I could I went to Droitwich and had massage and gentle exercise, and I very soon felt all right again. It is largely a question of nervous energy, grit, and determination.

My father had retired and was living at Droitwich when the fiftieth anniversary of his wedding came round, in 1907. To celebrate the event he and my mother held a large reception in the Kidderminster Town Hall, where they received many congratulations and handsome gifts. Their children gave them a gold loving-cup, which was handed to them at a luncheon party at my house, when thirty members of the family were present.

Twenty-seven years later, in 1934, my wife and I celebrated our own golden wedding by having a family dinner party at home. We also received many congratulations and beautiful gifts. References to both these Golden Weddings were made in the Lancet and the British Medical Journal.

CHAPTER V

SOME OF OUR ASSISTANTS

Duties of an assistant. Treatment of a fracture. A curious eye. Delirium tremens.
A so-called total abstainer. A black eye. Havana cigars.

I had sixteen years' experience of assistants myself and I have known many assistants to other members of the profession. Some of them are excellent, but others are dangerous in more ways than one. Most of them have to be taught by their principals, who at the same time have to pay them for their services, which seems rather an unfair arrangement. Many of the duties of an assistant may be described as of minor importance. Dispensing and the pricing of drugs, the filling in of certificates, and the treatment of minor ailments are apt to be disdained. A man who has recently passed his final examination is sometimes overwhelmed with the idea of his own importance and resents being taught details by a principal whom he looks upon as an old fossil in the country, but who probably knows more about general practice than all the hospital teachers put together. This bears out my view that the old system of apprenticeship cannot be surpassed.

The first assistant we had was an Irishman who had been a gold medallist at his hospital. He was a strange youth, whose Christian name was John. Shortly after his arrival one of my brothers introduced himself to him and asked him what his name was, meaning, of course, his surname. "Jack," he said. "Haven't you got any other name?" asked my brother. "No, it's just plain Jack," was the reply, and 'plain Jack' was the name he went by for the rest of his term with us. One night soon after he came I sent him up to the Workhouse to put up a simple fracture of a woman's forearm. When I arrived the next morning I found the patient's arm was extremely swollen and painful. I took off the bandages and then saw, to my horror and amazement, that 'plain Jack' had applied the splint with the pads outside and the wood next to the poor old woman's tissues. When I admonished him for this he tried to argue that he was right. He did not argue long. However, he was sober and had no vices, and he learnt some useful lessons during the year or two he was with us.

One of the best assistants we ever had was a Scotsman. He was a total abstainer and he did his work excellently, but he had a cast in his one eye, which gave him a peculiar appearance. One does not like to be too inquisitive and stare at people too much, but I had my suspicions about that eye. This man had been with us for some few months when there was an epidemic of influenza; he was laid up and I went to see him. When I knocked at his door I heard him jump out of bed and I was just in time to see him pick up something from the dressing-table and clap it into his eyelids - an artificial eye. This assistant stayed with us until he married and he did exceedingly well afterwards.

Another Irishman we had was quite a good man for the first five or six months, until he had to attend a patient suffering from delirium tremens; within a few days he was practically in the same condition himself. It is strange that this should have sent him off; he had evidently been a drunkard who had reformed. I could tell by the smell of his breath that he was drinking our tinctures. It would have been too dangerous to keep him, so I instantly paid him off and dismissed him.

Having had some experience with drunkards we resolved to try to get a total abstainer. An Irishman from Dublin applied for the post, stating that he was a total abstainer, and we engaged him. He arrived late one night and as I was unwell I did not see him that night. When he came in next morning I went to talk to him. I thought his breath smelt of alcohol, but I did not want to judge him unjustly so I waited and watched. His hands shook a great deal while he was making up the medicines. I walked to his rooms and questioned his landlady about him. "Oh," she said, "he was very drunk when he arrived. He put his feet on the grate and burnt the soles off his new shoes. He had a big dose of brandy before he got up and a pint of beer for his breakfast." Of course we could not keep him. When I told him he must go he begged and prayed me to give him another chance. I told him that I personally should have been quite willing to give him twenty chances, but I dared not do it because the lives of other people would be at stake; it would be criminal for me to allow him to continue at his job. I gave him enough money to pay his fare back home and he went to the station.

A week or two later his brother wrote to me from Dublin to ask if I could tell him what had become of his unfortunate brother. I did not know what had happened, but I gathered that he had been a drunkard before; his people had made him sign the pledge, got him a complete new outfit and sent him off to us, and he got drunk on the way. This sort of thing so often happens.

We had another man from Ireland, a champion athlete, a great burly fellow over six feet in height. He was all right at first, but after he had been with us a short time he began frequenting public-houses and behaving in a manner that was not in accordance with our ideas of respectability, so I made up my mind that I must get rid of him. I was rather frightened of this, however, because a few years before an assistant employed by my father and his partner, when reproved by the latter, knocked him down and blacked his eye. This called forth a paragraph in the next week's local newspaper headed "When doctors differ they fight to decide." So I poked my head round the door of the man's room, told him he had got to go and sent him his money when he went to have his supper.

Another assistant my father had had objected very much to the partner and was always saying what he was going to do to him. His one great idea was to let the pig loose in the garden, and he actually did this the night before he left. I looked upon him as rather a simpleton. For instance, when going to football matches, garden parties, and so on, he always had an ample provision of the very best Havana cigars with which he supplied us all freely. We thought it was a pity he should smoke such good cigars, so we bought some penny ones with which we used to present him. He would smoke these penny cigars and dilate upon then, their beauty, the perfect aroma, and so on, while we were smoking his Havanas and laughing up our sleeves. But I fancy he had the laugh on his side after all, because after he had left my father and his partner found that the Havana cigars had been ordered from their druggist and put down on their bill, and they had to pay for them. The assistant could not be found.

49

CHAPTER VI

CONVEYANCES

A pony-trap. Horse dealing. A trick of falling down. A millionaire owner. A carriage accident. White-legged horses. Van horses. A high-stepper. Age of horses. Legacy of horse. Another carriage accident. A hunt and a Jump. My first motor-car. A night drive. Return to horses. Cars again. Sale of a car. Age of a car. Cost of motoring. Motoring in the war years. Motor accidents.

The first conveyance I ever had was a pony-trap. I drove it myself and a little boy in buttons used to sit beside me. One of my earliest experiences with it was that when going down a hill one frosty day the pony spread-eagled and the little boy went head over heels out of the trap over him. Fortunately neither boy nor pony was hurt.

I have had a great many horses in my time and I have come to the conclusion that horse dealing is about the most dishonourable business in the world. I doubt if even a saint could be honest over it. My first horse was a very handsome cob. He had an unhappy knack of falling down without any warning. I might be driving along quite comfortably when all of a sudden down he went. I had to get rid of this animal and I knew his good looks would probably sell him, so I advertised him for sale. Several people answered the advertisement and the horse was sent over to the other side of Birmingham to be shown to a gentleman who wanted him for his wife to drive. My man rode him there and he actually fell down on the way; but the man brought only the saddle and bridle back with him, for they had bought the horse. Of course it would have been bad business, but I cannot help feeling that it would have been more in accordance with my views if I had written and told the applicants about the horse before they bought him.

I heard of a horse that was for sale in the Midlands. The owner was a millionaire who was known to my family, though not to myself. I went over to his place to look at the horse. He was a beautiful creature, a bay with four white legs and he looked as if he would be worth from £150 to £200. I had taken my man with me, a very shrewd horsy man who had been with a horse-dealer. He examined the horse thoroughly, then had him out and drove him about in the park. The coachman, who was a very grand gentleman, gave us every information about him, except the price. He said it would be necessary for me to see his master about that. I had a very pleasant interview with the old gentleman, who reminded me that he knew my father and others in my family. "Now what do you think of the horse? Will he suit you?" he said. "Yes," I replied, "I think he would suit me very well, but I doubt if I can afford to buy him." The old gentleman said he had sent the horse up to Tattersall's a month before and bought him in for £130. Then he had sent him to a repository in Birmingham and bought him in there for £90. I thought to myself that if the horse was worth as much as that there was not much chance of my getting him. However, the owner said, "I am so friendly with your family that you can have the horse at your own price. I have plenty of horses without him. Would £40 suit you as the price?" I could not afford £40 at that time, and on my suggesting £20 the old gentleman at once said, "I shall be delighted to let you have him for £20," and I had him. My man rode the horse home and before he got there he found out what was the matter with him. He was a confirmed jibber and I was soon glad to take a £10 note for him. I never complained to the millionaire, but for my own satisfaction I wrote to the Birmingham repository and ascertained that there had been no bid for the horse and he had been bought in for £20.

I must have had more than a hundred horse deals in my time and I came to the conclusion that the best plan for me was to buy my horses under the hammer and take my chance. Certainly I ran the risk of getting my neck broken and I once had a very narrow escape. I had a pair of horses that I had bought at a repository. One morning I was driving in the Victoria when, near the top of a very winding hill, a white and very silent motor-car hove in sight. The horses were terrified and swung round; as they did so I heard the pole snap, and I knew what was likely to happen. I got out of the carriage and saw the horses prancing and kicking. Being of a slight physical build I knew it was useless for me to go to their heads; I could only stand and look on. Ultimately my man fell off the box, fortunately unhurt. The horses set off full gallop down the hill with the carriage loose behind them. After they had got round the first corner we heard a most terrific crash. We picked up rug, whip, lamps and so on with which the road was strewn and started down the hill.

When we reached the scene of the crash we found the Victoria upside down, the axles bent so that it would be impossible to wheel it, and the two horses underneath it as if an extinguisher had been put on the top of them. Fortunately a number of labourers were working near and they came and lifted the carriage off the horses so that we could free them. One of them was unhurt; the other had cuts on her forehead and her hind-quarters. We took her home and I sewed up the cuts; the other horse I was driving in the afternoon. A curious thing about this accident is that in spite of all the damage done to the carriage in the smash, when everything else was broken, a glass aspirator bottle and the aspirating instruments, which were in a box in the front of the carriage, remained intact.

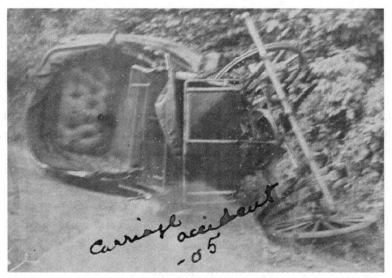

Victoria carriage accident – 1905

Another curious thing is that I had that morning arranged to take a rather infirm old aunt out in the carriage with me. Fortunately for her, something happened at the last moment to prevent her from going. She would almost certainly have been killed.

Here is a traditional saying about horses with white legs:

> "One: ride him for your life;
> Two: buy him for your wife;
> Three: try him;
> Four: don't buy him."

Though I do not believe in such superstitions it is a curious fact that nearly every horse I bought that had four white legs went wrong in some way or other. I once bought a beautiful chestnut with four white legs. He had been a hunter and was so handsome that my father took a great fancy to him. I let my father have him and within a month the horse was dead from a strangulated intestine. I once bought for a small sum of money a pair of horses that I saw in a van; at that time we were exceedingly busy and were short of horses. We drove one of them for twenty-five or twenty-six years, and she lived to be thirty-seven. We could not give her too much to do; she was a beautiful free easy-going mare worth her weight in gold.

I had another wonderful creature, a high-stepping mare over sixteen hands high. She could do a mile in three minutes comfortably; one day I drove her four miles in 12½ minutes. They laughed at me when I brought her home and said she would knock herself to pieces in twelve months. I drove her for ten years and sold her for twice what I had given for her. She was offered for sale again later; I sent my man to buy her and pensioned her off, putting her with a farmer where she lived in peace. The same thing had happened in the case of the horse that lived to be thirty-seven. Horses live to be quite old if they are properly cared for. I saw one once that was sixty-eight years old and I have read of one that was over ninety.

Strange stories are told about horses and it is not wise to believe all of them, but those I relate are all true. In 1898 an aunt of mine died and left me her horse, the harness, two carriages a Brougham and a Victoria and

£1,000. My father wanted me to have the whole lot sold and said I must not keep the horse because he was so dangerous. My aunt had talked to me about this before she died. She said that anybody to whom animals were bequeathed should keep them and take care of them, and I agreed with her. Nothing would have induced me to sell that horse.

The chief thing against him was that he was afraid of pigs; if he saw one in the road he would run away and upset the carriage. As this is partly a market town and there are often pigs about my old father was naturally rather alarmed. The day the horse arrived I had the saddle put on him and rode him myself. I had my man with me on another horse. I rode him out into the country, took him to a farm and rode him right up to the pigsty; he took no more notice of the pigs than if they had been flies. I never had any trouble with him afterwards and I kept him until he died.

On one occasion I was going out to do an operation in a village ten miles away. I had my father-in-law with me. Suddenly before I knew where I was my mare was on the ground and I was thrown out. Fortunately my father-in-law, being heavy, remained in the carriage. When I had picked myself up I found that one shaft of the buggy was broken, the mare was badly cut in the knees and there was a big flap of flesh hanging down from one of them. It would have been quite impossible for me to drive her on; I had an appointment to meet another doctor in less than half an hour and I had two miles to go on foot. So I took my bags out of the carriage, threw my overcoat in and told the old gentleman he must get some men to help him and do the best he could until I got back, but he must be sure to send a telegram home for another carriage.

I arrived in time to do the operation and the patient sent me back to where I had left the old gentleman. I found him comfortably ensconced in the parlour of the public-house, where he had ordered tea, poached eggs, ham and various other delicacies. He had had to send a man to walk four miles to take the telegram, so that it was very uncertain when we should get relief. In fact, the second horse and carriage with my man did not arrive until between 9 and 10 o'clock at night. Then we had to get the injured horse home. That was the only day in the whole course of my experience of over forty-one years (at that time) that I failed to see

55

everybody I had intended to see before I finished work for the day. When we got the mare home I sewed up her knee. The big flap that was hanging had to have ten or twelve stitches in it, dressings, bandages, and a knee-cap strapped over it. When they went to feed her and look after her the next morning she had got the dressings all off and had eaten the flap! In spite of that she got quite well and we were able to drive her for many years afterwards.

When one of my brothers was home from New Zealand he asked me to take him out riding. In the course of our ride we came across the foxhounds. My brother was very anxious to join in the hunt, but as I had no experience of such things I could not do so and I told him he would have to go by himself. They were going through a wood at the time, riding along a path I knew quite well. I decided to go with them through this path and leave my brother at the other end. We had to ride in single file; there would be perhaps about fifty horsemen and women. When we got about halfway along the path I saw to my horror that the horses in front of me were all jumping. A tree had fallen across the path and they were enjoying the jump. Worse still, the horse of the man just in front of me refused the jump; the man came off and they both tumbled down a bank on the left-handside. Thinking it would be my turn next, I let my mare go and held on to the saddle and fortunately I got over safely. I think that was my one and only jump, and that was my experience of hunting.

In the early days of motoring, about 1903, my brother was very anxious to sell me a motor-car, but I was not very much enamoured of them. He came over one Sunday afternoon from Cheltenham in a car and wanted to take me for a run in it. He said, "Of course you would probably have some difficulty in learning to drive, but when once you have learnt you will find a car is a great comfort." I sat by him in the car and very soon said to him, "Well now, you get out of that driving-seat and I will drive," and I drove fourteen miles without any difficulty or any instruction. I was so pleased at this that I gave my brother an order for a car, and three weeks later it arrived.

Mine was the first car in the borough; it was an Oldsmobile. It was before the days of numbering cars; when that became the rule I got an early number, AB10, which I kept, on different cars, for thirty-three

56

years. I got rid of my horses and started motoring regularly, and a most wretched time I had! We never went out without something going wrong and I had great difficulty in getting through my work.

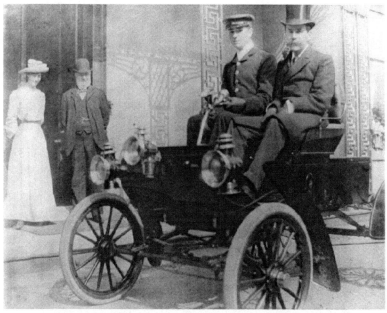

Lionel, with chauffeur H Teale, in his first car - 1903 Oldsmobile
Recorded as an "American motorised dog-cart" in the County Records
Courtesy of Timothy Wadsworth

On one occasion I was coming home after midnight and when we got to the top of a hill I found that neither of the brakes would act. We had two or three steep hills to negotiate on the way home. Not being physically strong myself, I knew I could not hold the car on the hill, and I knew that my man could not do it either. At that time I was not learned enough in motoring to know that by putting the car into low gear you can go slowly down the hills. I said to my man, "Well, the only thing is for me to drive and you to get up alongside and say the prayers." I suppose he did so, for we got home safely.

After various irritating and dangerous experiences with cars I decided to go back to horses. By the time I had the carriage accident already described cars had become more reliable, so I thought I had better try one again. This time I had a Clement Talbot.

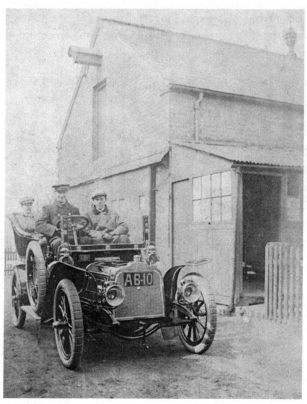

12 – 16 Clement Talbot
~1909

After this car had had a good deal of wear I advertised it in the Auto-Car. The advertisement brought me letters from several garages in London, informing me that they had many customers asking for cars like mine and assuring me that they would be able to sell it to very good advantage if I would let them have it on view. The car was sent to one of these places and I heard no more about it for some time. I became rather anxious, and still more so when I heard by accident that the car had been seen in another garage. Eventually I found out that the people to whom I had sent it had sold it and spent the money. I got into touch with the Police and the Public Prosecutor, and the miscreants were brought to book. It came out in the Court that they had cheated dozens of people in the same way. When I attended to give evidence I was very much amused at the detective. I asked him when I could have my car back. He replied, "Well, Sir, you can't have it at all. If it had been stolen you could have it, but this is a misdemeanour, not a theft, and you can't have it." I could only say to him, "The law is an ass," and we had a good laugh over it.

People do not realise in these days all the troubles we went through before the cars were so perfected as they are now. I was often accused of extravagance because I kept three cars. I began with one, then I had two, until I found that in order to keep myself efficient and able to give constant service I must have three, because one or two of them might be in dock at any time.

Some people say it is necessary to buy a new car every year. I feel satisfied in my own mind that if a good car is properly looked after[2] it will run for 100,000 miles. The age of a car is estimated by the number of years it has been in use, but as a matter of fact the age of a car is really the number of miles it has run and the way in which it has been taken care of.

There is great diversity of opinion as to the cost of motoring. Most people make themselves believe, or profess to believe, that motoring is cheaper than horses and carriages. It is true that a motor widens your sphere of activity but, having had a very long and varied experience of both, I can unhesitatingly assert that the cost of motoring is nearly double that of a carriage and a pair of horses. I find that when people are talking about the cost of motoring they usually omit certain important items of the expense; for instance, the interest on the money the car cost, and depreciation, which on a £500 car amounts to about £100 a year.

If a man has no chauffeur he saves the wages, but he often has to be satisfied to go about in a filthy car and the neglect of his car and his engine probably costs him in the long run a considerable proportion of the sum that he would have spent on an efficient chauffeur. I regard myself as a very fortunate man in having possessed such an excellent servant as I had for over forty years. He was originally my coachman and

---

[2] See Addenda 5.6 & 5.7

then became my chauffeur. His son now holds that office and is in the twentieth year of his service with me.

During the war I had experience of the miseries that must be suffered by those who are at the mercy of inefficient chauffeurs, for though my man had a large family and was by no means physically strong he was determined to join up. Eventually a lady patient came to my rescue; not only did she drive me, but she provided her own car. On two or three occasions for several weeks at a time she did everything for me, looking after the car as well as driving me. But except when with her, I never was happy or safe in motoring until I got my own man back.

I have had several motor accidents, but fortunately no very serious ones. They chiefly consisted in running over dogs - a very unpleasant experience, but I consider it is better than risking the lives of human beings in order to avoid injury to animals.

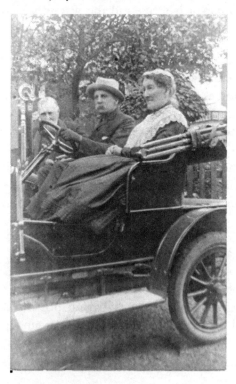

Lionel with his wife and father ~1912

CHAPTER VII

VISITS TO GERMANY

Visit to Berlin, 1890. Koch's tuberculin. Interpreter. Virchow and the Charité Hospital. Patients under discipline. Sewage farm. Homburg, 1908. Arrangements for reception and entertainment. Springs. Toast of Homburg Medical Society. Warnings of impending war with France. Baths. Zander Institute. Frankfort and Nauheim. Königstein. "The Merry Widow." Banquet at Ritter's Park Hotel.

In 1882 Robert Koch discovered the bacillus of tuberculosis[3]. In 1890 members of the profession from all over the world were flocking to Berlin to learn about the tuberculin that he then put forward as a cure for the disease. I visited Berlin in company with a friend and colleague, and we spent a most interesting week there. We arrived at 11.30 on a Saturday night and found that all the hotels were crowded; we were fortunate enough to secure the last room that was vacant in the Hôtel Continental. We were then faced with the difficulty that we could not speak German, so in order to gain access to the various hospitals and get the best information possible we engaged an interpreter. He was a very intelligent man and for the sum of 20 Marks a day he proved an invaluable help to us.

The hospitals in Berlin began work at about 8 o'clock in the morning, and our interpreter arrived at our hotel at 7.30 to take us wherever we wished to go. The first morning, a Sunday, he took us to the Charité Hospital, but he was told at the porter's office that we could not be admitted on a Sunday. I was not to be done in that way, so we waited until some students went in and we got into the ward with them. We

---

[3] See Addendum 3.2

watched the injections of tuberculin and our interpreter explained to us the chief remarks of the physicians. One of them offered me the syringe to give some injections. In those days they were not so particular about asepsis as we are now, but I felt it would not be right for me to give the injections so I politely refused.

Sir James Paget had given me a letter of introduction to Professor Virchow and we visited him at his private house. The next morning he met us at the Charité to show us his pathological department and we spent a most interesting time with him. At that time there were over 1,000 beds in the hospital and the patients appeared to be well cared for and happy. Virchow told us that they were under strict discipline and were obliged to submit to any treatment, operative or any other, that was recommended for them. This is a great contrast to the methods adopted in our own country. All the bodies were subject to post-mortem examination, and the work was thoroughly well done.

We also had an introduction to Koch and went to see him at his Pathological Institute but had not time for conversation with him. At all the hospitals we were received with great cordiality and treated with the utmost politeness.

Our interpreter accompanied us everywhere, took us to suitable restaurants for lunch and to places of amusement in the evening. One afternoon we had an interesting visit to the sewage farm, managed by the municipality. The work there was chiefly done by men and women vagrants who, when committed for begging or minor crimes, were sentenced to a term of detention at the sewage farm. They were housed and fed there and at the end of their period of detention they were given a sum of money representing wages for the work they had done. It seemed to me a very excellent and practical arrangement to make use of the labour of these people. Sometimes there were as many as 500 of them at work; and the farm paid a dividend.

In June, 1908, I spent a week at Homburg as a guest of the Municipality and the Medical Society there. I was one of a party of between twenty and thirty medical men from this country. The arrangements made for our reception and entertainment were a conspicuous example of German thoroughness. We were met at the station and escorted to our various hotels. There we found on our dressing-tables a complete programme, printed in English, of the events arranged for the whole week of our stay; almost every hour was accounted for. The first night there was a reception at 9 p.m, at the Kurhaus. This was arranged on a system new to me and it reminded me of a whist drive. The large reception room contained many small tables. Each of us was conducted to a separate table, where two or three of our German colleagues were waiting to receive us. Every quarter of an hour a bell rang and we all changed tables. All our hosts wanted to become personally acquainted with us, and it seemed to me that this was a good way of doing it.

The next morning we had an address from Dr. Hoeber on the Homburg cure treatment and then we inspected the bath establishments. It was Dr. Hoeber who always attended King Edward when he had treatment at Homburg. In the evening there was a banquet at the Kurhaus by invitation of the Directors. We English doctors were all more or less unknown to one another, but I had made friends with one from London in the railway train, and we remained friends until he died some years later. He had a very distinguished appearance and he had been approached by some of the others about replying to the toast of the English doctors that was proposed at the banquet. He insisted that I should be the one to do this. I did not mind in the least, for I was accustomed to and rather fond of speaking in public, but I could not imagine how he knew this. However, I responded to the toast, and I was called upon to speak on several occasions afterwards, one being at a dinner given to us by the Homburg Medical Society at the Grand Hotel, when it fell to my lot to propose the toast of the Society. They had a curious arrangement of interspersing the toasts with the various courses. I had to get up after the fish course. In the light of subsequent events it may be of some interest to record my speech, which ran as follows:

> "I rise with great diffidence to propose success to the Homburg Medical Society. Your town possesses many advantages. Its situation and natural beauty are a source of admiration, and this natural beauty is increased by artificial improvements that are not exaggerated to the extent of spoiling Nature. It has various springs of therapeutic value suitable for the treatment of divers complaints. It has baths and appliances of many kinds, all of them

constructed on the best principles and all of them kept in splendid condition and thoroughly up to date. It has two forms of mud, and if they are as valuable in treatment as they are repulsive to look at they must indeed be a great possession. It has a climate which is most invigorating. Added to all these advantages it enjoys to a very large extent the blessing of good government. In your Kurdirektor you have the perfect man for such a position. Your Mayor and Corporation, if I may judge by results, are very capable officers, and your Medical Society contains men of high scientific attainments.

"I have long been aware that you are great organisers, from your Emperor, for whom I have a profound admiration, downwards. Your Medical Society is evidence of this. Omnes sapientes decet conferre et fabulari. It has been a great privilege to confer with you, and the willingness with which you have placed your knowledge and your time at our disposal is fully appreciated by us.

"We on our side of the Channel fully appreciate the debt which our profession owes to your country. We rejoice with you in the possession of such stalwart sons as Rudolph Virchow and Professor Koch, whose names will remain for all time.

"In our profession we can claim, I think, to be more broadminded than the average man. We are not affected by temporary political or racial differences, but we are bound together by bonds which nothing can sever. Tonight we grasp the hand of friendship which you hold out to us. Such meetings as this must tend to increase our entente cordiale, as you happily expressed it in your invitation to us.

"Is it too much to hope that it may be the harbinger of a far greater tie, an entente which shall bind our two countries together, not only for their own mutual advantage, but for the benefit of the whole of the civilised world? God grant it may be so!

"In conclusion I have to thank you for your princely hospitality and your continuous kindness and courtesy. We wish every success to your Society. Floreat! I desire to couple with this toast the name of your learned President, Dr......."

This speech was received with great enthusiasm. I was afraid one man was going to embrace me; luckily he just stopped short of that! I was favoured with invitations to lunch and breakfast at the private houses of Dr. Hoeber and other prominent doctors in Homburg. One of them told me that there would soon be war between Germany and France, but that England would not be in it. He asked me if I had noticed numbers on the railway carriages, which I had done. He said these numbers referred to the soldiers they were to carry and that everything was arranged; all the railway servants knew exactly what they had to do and the moment the Emperor pressed the button the war machine would work. Germany would be able to place half a million of men on the frontier within a week and a million within a fortnight. This was in 1908; I did not think much about it then, but I have thought of his words many times since. When the war did break out the information he had given me made me think that Paris would fall within a week of the outbreak. It is a miracle that it did not.

Every morning I was in Homburg I got up at 5 o'clock and had a two hours' walk into the country before we met at the springs at 7 a.m. The bath establishments were all beautifully kept, the baths were very fine and the attendants very well dressed in livery. There were all kinds of baths - mud, effervescent, Russian, Turkish, etc. The mud pack was horrible-looking stuff.

We were taken to Frankfurt to see the house where Goethe was born, and to Nauheim to visit the baths. We also inspected the Homburg Hospital and the open-air and sun-baths that had recently been established on the outskirts of the town in a field of about 5 or 6 acres.

One day we inspected the Zander Institute. This is provided with all kinds of machinery for performing the various movements of the body and exercising the muscles. Amongst the appliances was an artificial horse, and I shall never forget the sight of a portly dignitary of the English church jogging up and down on it; he looked to me as if he would burst.

65

We were taken to Königstein, a beautiful place in the Taunus mountains, where people sometimes go from Homburg for an after-cure. We went to a special performance of "The Merry Widow" at the theatre, where the Emperor's box was placed at our disposal. On Sunday we attended the English church; then we had lunch at the private house of one of the doctors and afterwards went to an "At Home"; in the evening the proprietors of the Ritter's Park Hotel, where King Edward used to stay, entertained us at a truly magnificent banquet.

When we left Homburg, after having enjoyed a most agreeable and instructive holiday, our hosts saw us off at the station. I had not spent five hours in bed any night of that week, yet I never felt better in my life than when I came back. The air was most invigorating and suited me to perfection.

CHAPTER VIII

HOLIDAYS

Definition of work. Definition of holiday. Housewife's need of holiday. Rest and sleep. Two medical opinions. Excesses on holiday. Risks. Anticipation, realisation, and contemplation. Bicycle tours. Children and holidays. Advantage of personal knowledge of holiday resorts. Channel Islands. Continental holiday. St. Bernard Hospice. War atmosphere in France. Lack of refinement abroad.

Work was once defined to me as an escape from boredom, which I consider a better definition than those usually found in dictionaries. I maintain that any effort, physical or mental, is work. Surely the professional cricketer works; the professional golfer, the huntsman, the chess-player, and many others, also work. Yet if we were to indulge in these pursuits we should consider that we were playing.

My definition of a holiday is: an escape from one's daily occupation. I believe that when people become so bored with their daily occupation that they long for a respite it is a benefit to them to have a change of occupation for a time. A turn of rowing, golfing, or hunting may be very beneficial to a surgeon, and it is a pity the professional golfer cannot take a turn at medicine for his holiday.

Of all the possible occupations, I can think of none that is more likely to be wearisome than that of a housewife. I have always maintained that men have by far the best of life. It is the women-folk who bear the greatest burdens, but unfortunately men do not always realise this. The housewife would benefit by a change more than once a year; it would be good for her health, good for her temper, and good for her husband.

In the question of holidays, as in regard to all other questions, individuals vary. Some men - and I am happy to be one of them - are so infatuated, may I say, with their occupation that they never want to leave it and they do not get stale at it. I think this applies more particularly to a profession like my own, which holds so much variety. I could not sit on an office stool posting ledgers day after day, year in and year out, without pining for diversion. My own work provides me with constant changes. No two cases are alike and the study of their infinite variety is so fascinating to me that I have been unable to tear myself away for the last thirty years. I cannot help feeling that my own experience negatives the present-day fetish that an annual holiday is necessary for everybody. In olden days people did not have so much. I quite admit that an annual holiday is agreeable to most people, and in some few cases it may even be desirable, but that is a very different thing from being necessary. When it is said to be necessary, presumably it is from a health point of view.

I suppose nobody can work continuously. All of us take periods of rest. These periods are chiefly occupied in sleep, and the amount of sleep that individuals require varies considerably. The average time would be, I suppose, seven or eight hours, but there are instances on record where men of great mental power, who used their brains to an enormous extent, needed considerably less. The great John Hunter, for example, used to sleep for only four hours out of the twenty-four. A relative of mine habitually had only four hours of sleep every night; he told me that when he went to bed he put his head down on his pillow, went instantly to sleep, and remained absolutely oblivious of everything until he woke four hours later. Many people, like myself, do not know what it means to go to sleep immediately they lie down. They lie awake for an hour or two, wake several times in the night, and always dream when asleep. Their brain probably never goes to sleep. It is understandable that people who sleep more soundly than others can do with a shorter period of sleep. Most people have the Sunday for rest, and a half-holiday on Saturday or on some other day in the week as well. During recent years this half-holiday has been increased to a whole day for many trades, which in my opinion is a very doubtful benefit.

It is a question whether it is more desirable to have short, intermittent rests or an occasional orgy of rest. In my opinion temporary and well-distributed periods of relaxation are more beneficial; for instance, two or three hours at golf or tennis, billiards or cards, gardening or carpentering.

68

I am certain that orgies of rest often result in disaster for the people who indulge in them.

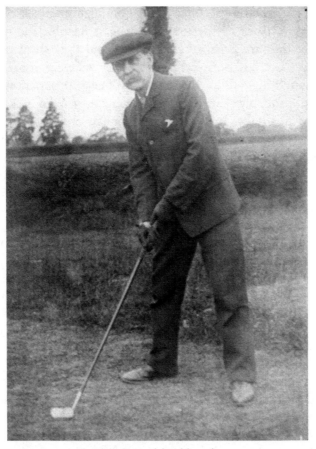

Lionel practising his swing

I once discussed the question of holidays with two eminent medical men in London. One of them urged me to go on a voyage; he said that a long holiday was the finest investment in the world; even if it cost £500 or £1,000 it was well worth it. I listened to him quite politely but did not take his advice. The other one asked me what I thought about holidays. He was a canny Scot and wanted to find out my own views before he offered me any advice. I told him I did not believe in holidays. "My dear fellow," he said, "you make a great mistake; holidays are the finest things in the world for us. If it were not for holidays I should have nothing to

69

do in the winter. I spend all my winters in trying to cure people of illnesses they have contracted while on their holidays."

Most people when away on a holiday indulge in excesses of various kinds, which must be very detrimental to their health. I do not mean to insinuate that they are immoral or drunken; but they sleep too much or too little, they eat far more or far less, they take far more or far less exercise, than when following their ordinary occupation. All such excesses are probably harmful. Moreover, they take risks that they ordinarily do not, take, by travelling in public conveyances, staying in unhealthy places, and so on. Numbers of people have contracted enteric fever through getting into insanitary places or drinking impure milk or water while on holiday. We are not so likely to do this at home, because there things are more under our own control; we can look after our own sanitary arrangements and our own food and drink.

In spite of all risks and drawbacks I admit that visits to places of interest are sometimes both agreeable and advantageous. The pleasure of a holiday is threefold: anticipation, realisation, contemplation. Still a further joy, and perhaps not the least, is the joy of coming home again when the holiday is over.

Anticipation includes arrangements to be made for the household during our absence, decisions as to what we shall need to take with us, and so on. From a woman's point of view the planning and wearing of suitable and becoming clothes add greatly to the charm of a holiday, and it would be churlish to spoil her pleasure in this. A woman will try to persuade you that the purchase of new clothes for the holiday will be economical in the long, run, and she will probably succeed. There are plenty of people, of both sexes, who can always satisfy themselves that it is economical to buy anything that they specially desire.

The realisation sometimes does not quite come up to the anticipation, though it may occasionally exceed it. Sometimes people start cheerfully for a holiday and when they reach their destination find they cannot get lodgings and they have to suffer all sorts of discomforts. To be obliged to sleep on the esplanade or on a billiard-table, as I have known people do, is not my idea of an enjoyable holiday. If we are wise we shall not leave home unless we know beforehand that we shall be properly provided for.

The third and greatest joy, the joy that can never be taken away from us, is the contemplation, the remembrance of the beautiful scenery we have admired, of the interesting places we have visited, and of the pleasant circumstances connected with our holiday. No matter what misfortunes may befall us afterwards, we can always remember and re-live these agreeable experiences in our minds. Most people forget the disagreeable episodes, and those who remember them will find that they assume smaller proportions after the lapse of years. The happiest method of dealing with them is to try to derive some pleasure from them by thinking of the humorous aspect that most of them possess, though that side does not always occur to us until later.

Although I have not been away for a holiday for more than thirty years I think I have made a more thorough examination of our own country than most people have. If you want really to know a country there are few better ways of doing it than by making tours on a push-bicycle. In these days such a mode of progression is scoffed at; it must be motor-cars and motor-bicycles. Having travelled a good deal by both, I unhesitatingly assert that the motor vehicles convey you through the scenery far too quickly for you to enjoy its beauties; on the push-bicycle you can quietly meander along and when you come to any specially attractive spot you can get off your bicycle, sit down and give yourself time to observe and enjoy it thoroughly.

There are certain essentials if you want really to enjoy such a bicycle tour. First, you must have a congenial companion, and it must be thoroughly understood that the stronger rider must adapt his pace to that of the weaker one; otherwise the whole pleasure will be spoilt. Second, you must have a good make of machine, in thorough order and capable of completing the distance you propose to ride without any likelihood of a breakdown. Third, you should provide means of carrying your luggage with you. After various annoying experiences connected with luggage the friend who usually accompanied me in my tours devised a very excellent frame box, made of mahogany, and watertight. It locked up and, though not heavy, was large enough to carry a suit of clothes in addition to all the usual requirements, collars, cuffs, shaving materials,

71

hair-brushes, and extra socks and shirts. This box, with a hold-all behind containing one's night attire and an extra pair of boots, enabled us to frequent the best hotels in all the fashionable places and to go down to table d'hôte dinner feeling quite comfortable. I had a special suit made for such occasions, of a kind of silky serge, which was so light that I could almost have wrapped it up and put it in my pocket.

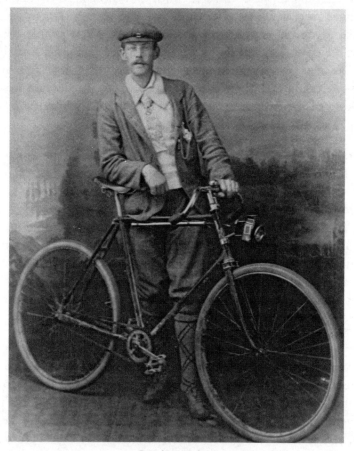

Brother Hubert

So far as children are concerned I hold the view that not only are holidays unnecessary for them but that the children in most instances are better at home. Parents would derive more benefit from their holidays if they left the children at home. Certainly the mother would; she should be free from the cares and anxieties of her children when she goes for her holiday, and it is not a holiday for her unless she is. Of course care must be taken to provide an efficient substitute to look after them at home. I would take children for holidays only when they are old enough to appreciate it, and as part of their education.

Before deciding where to go for a holiday people often consult their doctor, and it is a great advantage for him to have personal knowledge of a variety of health and pleasure resorts. If for no other reason, the cycle tours I have advocated are very valuable; and I would emphasise the importance of gaining a thorough knowledge of one's own country before going abroad. Those who spend their holidays at the same place year after year are not advancing their education, improving their minds, or enlarging their store of memories for future happy contemplation. It is a great advantage to go to as many different places as possible while you are young, because you then have so many more years of retrospective enjoyment.

I have ridden over England, Wales, Scotland, and Ireland, and there are few places on the coast that I have not visited, from Land's End to John o' Groat's, and from the Giants' Causeway to Killarney. All parts, of our islands have their own particular beauty and are well worth visiting, and in most of the towns there is excellent accommodation. If you want to go a little farther afield, from an economical point of view one of the best holidays is a visit to the Channel Islands. One of the charms of these islands is that they have such a variety of beautiful scenery.

In my young days I could not afford any expensive holiday, so I never went on the Continent. However, an opportunity arrived in 1889, when my father had a wealthy patient - a lady - who was ordered a trip on the Continent. It was necessary for her to have a medical attendant with her; I was offered the position for a month. I accepted it on condition that my wife should be allowed to go with us. A relative of the patient also went with us as her companion, so that she could sleep with her at night and generally look after her. We were to travel in the most luxurious way and stay at the best hotels, and the choice of the itinerary was left very largely to me, We had some varied experiences, not all pleasant ones, and saw some of the chief cities in Belgium, Germany, Switzerland, and France, and spent a night at the Hospice of St. Bernard. The monks make no charge to visitors. Their doors are ever open to the wayfarer, who is received, lodged and fed gratis. The question of what should be given in return for the hospitality is left to the generosity - or the meanness - of those who accept it. I had been reading that the average amount received in those days (this was in 1889) was something under 1 franc for each person for a night. How people can be so mean I cannot understand! But if they all had the same difficulty as I had in finding somewhere to deposit their money perhaps there is a little excuse for them if they gave nothing. I should think it took me quite an hour; eventually I found an alms-box in their church, and into that box I put the same amount of money as we should have paid at an hotel. Even that would be cheap when you think that everything had to be carried up some 8,000 feet, part of the way on the backs of ponies.

Even in those days I was struck by the military appearance of Strasburg. The streets positively bristled with bayonets and one felt that the future must bring war; it seemed to be in the atmosphere. In Paris again I was impressed with the feeling of impending war when I saw the Place de la Concorde with the statue representative of Strasburg decorated with wreaths to keep alive the remembrance of the Franco-German War and the losses it meant to France. What struck me very much on the Continent was the lack of refinement everywhere evidenced, even in the best hotels. No wonder the refinement of English people is a matter of comment outside their own country!

I was very glad to get back to London and to the good old English custom of a cut from the joint. The foreign food was all done up in a tasty kind of fashion, but I never knew what I was eating. The realisation of this continental holiday was no great joy, but the contemplation of it, the recollection of all the beautiful things and places we saw has been a constant source of pleasure to me ever since and I balance that against the discomfort we suffered at the time.

CHAPTER IX

THRIFT

Habits. Pocket-money. A student's living expenses. Saving out of income. Improvidence among working classes. Remedy. Exceptions to rule.

We are all creatures of habit. Many of our habits are formed in early life and it is very difficult to alter them later. The habit of careless spending of money is so easy to attain that special efforts should be made to prevent its formation and to inculcate the habit of thrift. There is no better way of fostering extravagance than to allow children a large amount of pocket-money, and for this the parents are responsible. Even if a boy is to be possessed of wealth and one of the objects of his education is to teach him to spend it, I feel that it would be an advantage if he were made to deny himself in his early years; he should be taught the responsibility of wealth and the happiness that can be obtained from the proper use of it.

The pocket-money my mother gave me was two-pence a week, and it remained the same until I left school at the age of sixteen. My allowance was then increased to two shillings a week, but out of this I had to provide my own boots, gloves, and neckties. I was fortunate in receiving some handsome tips from well-to-do relations and friends, but most of these sums were put into the bank to provide me with a capital.

Perhaps it was because I was precocious, I do not know, but my parents let me more or less into the secrets of their financial position. I accepted their explanation and my own reason forced me to believe that they were in financial difficulties, with a large and increasing family to bring up and educate. My affection for them was so profound that I felt it my duty to deny myself in every possible way in order to make things easier for them. I was honest enough to say, and I have often repeated,

75

that I would never have worked if my father had been a wealthy man. I should have chosen to live a life of sport. This too is a form of work, but it is not the work that earns one's daily bread; it is of little use to one's fellow-men, and it cannot in the long run bring the satisfaction that conscientious men and women desire above everything else in life.

I lived very economically when I was a student at St. Bartholomew's. People will not believe it when I tell them now, but I often spent only one penny on my lunch, because I could not afford two-pence, or thought I could not. The penny meant a glass of milk; if I spent two-pence, a bun was added to the milk. Two or three of us students lived together in lodgings in various places. At one time when three of us lived together we paid 30/- a week for our rooms, coals and lights. I was the housekeeper. I used to buy a piece of bacon, carry it home and have it boiled, so that we could have it cold for breakfast, with porridge and bread and butter. We had our frugal lunch at about 1 o'clock and were back home to a good meal at 5 o'clock; this would consist of a leg of mutton or a piece of beef, vegetables, a pudding, cheese, and a bottle of beer. Our living, including lodgings, cost us from £1 to 25/- a week each. I always did the catering and the carving, another man served the vegetables, and the third one rang the bell; it was an equal division of labour!

My later experience has convinced me that it is a very good thing for boys to be hard up when they are young. But however hard up they may be, I maintain that they should try to save something; they should attain the habit of living within their means. I had an interesting illustration of this some years ago. One morning a lady whom I was attending told me about one of her sons. She said: "That boy is in a situation hundreds of miles away; he earns only 35/- a week, he keeps himself, he pays for his own clothes and personal expenses and never asks us for a copper. Isn't he splendid?" "How much does he save?" I asked. Whereupon she exclaimed indignantly, "Save! I told you he only gets 35/- a week. How could you possibly expect him to save anything?" "Oh, I don't know," I said meekly, "I thought perhaps he might save something."

I went on my round and later in the morning another lady spoke to me in similar terms, telling me what a fine boy her son was. He was earning only 25/- a week, yet he kept himself entirely and never asked

76

his parents for a penny piece. Didn't I think him splendid? Of course I agreed, but I asked her also how much he saved. She too exclaimed indignantly, "Save! Out of 25/- a week! How could he?"

Now comparing these two stories it was obvious that the first boy might have saved 10/- a week. I had in my mind at the moment a friend of my own, who told me that during his training for the medical profession he never spent more than 13/6 a week on his living. He studied in Aberdeen, though he was not a Scotsman. It does not follow that if one man can live on this amount another can, but he might at least try to learn to do it. There is proof positive that it can be done.

Nearly forty years ago I was invited to preside at a dinner to celebrate the jubilee of a certain thrift society, which for fifty years had proved of great benefit to the working men and women in the town. I congratulated the members upon the success of their society and explained my own views on thrift: that a certain part of the regular income should be set aside as savings and put in the Post Office Savings Bank or invested in some reliable Government securities, not in any wild-cat schemes; the rest should be spent to the very best advantage. I tried to bring home to my hearers the fact that poor people are in many instances paying far more than the rich for the same things. For instance, poor people buy coal by the hundredweight, a much more costly way than buying it by the ton or by the load. I remember asking a man years ago how it was that he could afford to pay so much more for everything than I did. He was absolutely amazed when I explained to him that he was doing so. At that time I was buying beer at 1/- a gallon and he was paying four-pence a pint for his; that is, he was paying 2/8 a gallon for what I got for 1/-.

The cause of this sort of thing is usually said to be the want of capital. But is not improvidence often at the root of it? It is well known amongst collectors that if they fail to appear on the day that the amount they collect is due the money will be spent on something else. The average person seems to be incapable of putting money on one side. If working-class people would have a system of money-boxes and conscientiously put so much aside each week for coal and other necessaries they would then be able to buy these things on more advantageous terms. The same principle applies more or less to all classes of society.

Yet persistently as I preach the doctrine of thrift and urge everyone regularly to save some part of his income, however small, I cannot deny that there are exceptions to every rule, and I have sometimes felt obliged to advise patients that they must spend the whole of their income. These have always been patients who were dependent upon their salaries for a living, and whose constitutions made it essential for them to live under as comfortable conditions as possible if they were to be enabled to carry on their work.

CHAPTER X

CHAIRMANSHIPS

Membership of British Medical Association. Chairman of Worcester Division. National Health Insurance Scheme. Chairmen of Worcestershire and Herefordshire Branch of B.M.A. Complimentary dinner and presentation from Worcester Division, 1921. Story of a fur-lined coat. War work as Chairman of Local Medical Committee. Appeal to the public. Chairman of Local Emergency Committee, 1939. Chairman of Panel Committee. Complimentary dinner and presentation from Panel Committee, 1935. Thanks. Letter from Dr. Alfred Cox. Kidderminster Medical Society.

In the early years of my membership of the British Medical Association I was so fully occupied with my practice and with the medico-political and the scientific work of our local Medical Society that I seldom attended any of the meetings of the Association. It was therefore a great surprise to me when in the year 1910 I received from the Worcester Division of the British Medical Association a request that they might be allowed to nominate me as their Chairman. I acceded to this request and was elected Chairman.

My year of office was characterised by an enormous amount of work in connection with the establishment of the National Health Insurance Scheme. The year came to an end before the arrangements connected with the Insurance Act were completed. It was one of the Rules of the Association that no member should hold the position of Chairman for two years in succession, but this Rule was suspended to enable me to go on with the negotiations relating to the Insurance Act. After that piece of work was finished and the National Health Insurance Scheme had been established I was appointed Chairman of the Worcestershire and Herefordshire Branch of the British Medical Association.

I was again Chairman of the Worcester Division of the Association at two later periods, in the years 1915-16 and 1919-20. In the year 1921 the Division invited me to a complimentary dinner at Worcester, at which they presented me with a very handsome silver salver, bearing the following inscription: "Presented to J. Lionel Stretton, Esq. by members of the Worcester Division of the British Medical Association in recognition of his valued services and of the esteem in which he is held. January 20th, 1921."

In my speech of thanks I referred to the high ideals that had been set before me by my forbears and to the distinguished members of the profession with whom I had been intimately acquainted. In this connection I related the following story. When Mr. Balfour was Prime Minister he sent an emissary to a certain eminent physician to offer him a knighthood. The physician sent his thanks and said he did not want a knighthood. Mr. Balfour thought he expected a baronetcy and sent to offer him one. Again the physician expressed his thanks but declined the honour. "Well," said Mr. Balfour, "go and ask him what he does want." "Please thank Mr. Balfour and say that I should like a fur-lined coat," was the physician's reply. He had the fur-lined coat. I went on to say that I had been much interested in the work of the Division; I paid a tribute to the services of the Secretary; and I appealed to all the members, and more especially the younger ones, to be regular attendants at the meetings so that they might have a voice in framing the policy of the Association.

During the Great War I was Chairman of the Local Medical Committee for the County of Worcester. This Committee had to decide which of the doctors should join up when extra calls were made for the services of medical men in the county. The Chairmanship was a very difficult position to hold and it brought me into contact with most of the members of the profession in the County. It seems remarkable that I was able to carry on this work throughout the whole period of the war without, so far as I am aware, making a single enemy among them. I always explained to any of them who came to see me that in deciding who was to join up the Committee could not give any weight to personal reasons. If a man had an invalid wife, or was in such a financial position that his going away would ruin him, it would not have the slightest effect upon the Committee's decision. The one and only point we had to consider was which man could best be spared, so as to afford the least possibility of depriving the general public of the efficient medical service they had a right to expect.

A letter, signed by myself and by the Honorary Secretary of the Committee, was published in the local press in March, 1916. It directed public attention to the difficulties under which the medical profession was labouring owing to the absence of so many of its members on war service; it offered suggestions whereby those remaining in civil practice might be better enabled to support the extra strain thrown upon them, without depriving their patients of necessary care and attention; and it appealed for loyalty to ensure that those on active service might find on their return that their practices had not suffered from their absence.

I believe that not one of the men from this district lost his life during the war. One man from Kidderminster won the M.C.

At the present time (1939) I hold a position similar to that I occupied during the war: the Chairmanship of the Local, Emergency Committee for the Worcestershire and Bromsgrove Area.

I have never been a panel practitioner, but in 1912 I was elected Chairman of the County of Worcester Local Medical and Panel Committee; I have held that position continuously, having been re-elected every two years, and I still hold it. Few things in my career have given me more satisfaction than the honour that was paid me on November 29th, 1933, when this Committee gave me a complimentary dinner and presentation at an hotel in Kidderminster to celebrate my twenty-first year of office as Chairman. There was a large gathering of medical men representative of all parts of the County. The present consisted of a silver dessert service of exceptionally beautiful design and workmanship, and it bears the following inscription: "Presented by the County of Worcester Local Medical and Panel Committee as a token of esteem, regard and affection, to John Lionel Stretton, who had been their Chairman continuously for 21 years, July, 1933."

The last part of my speech of thanks was as follows:-

"In speaking of the work that we have done together on the Panel Committee I should like to acknowledge the loyal support

81

you have given me. You have always upheld any decision I have been obliged to make. You have been an easy team to drive, and our Chief Whip, the Secretary, is so well versed in the National Insurance Act, and so keenly interested in the Panel Committee, that my duties have been very light.

"I can only say, Thank you, for your kindness to me tonight, but I assure you that these two words mean more than I can express. Believe me, I shall never forget it. The contemplation of it will cheer me in the years to come, and your beautiful present will be one of my most cherished possessions. When the time comes for it to be handed down in my family as an heirloom I can only hope that it may be a stimulus to others to try to play the game, as I have tried to play it. Thank you!"

Almost equally gratifying to me was the following letter I received soon afterwards from Dr. Alfred Cox, formerly Secretary of the British Medical Association, with whom I had had many dealings, and some controversy, in the past:-

"I have just read the account in last week's B.M.J. of the presentation to yourself and I should like to congratulate you, and still more your colleagues, on this sign of appreciation of long and loyal service.

"There is nobody who has more cause to appreciate the gratitude of his friends than I have, and like you I believe there is nothing of which a man may be more justly proud than the recognition of his own people amongst whom and for whom he has worked, and who know him better than most.

"I have known you for very many years as a hard worker, a strong fighter, and the very devil to move if you had come to a conclusion as to the right course to take. I hope increasing years will never diminish your interest in the affairs of your profession and that you may have good health to enjoy the respect of your fellows."

In 1893 the Kidderminster Medical Society was formed, with my father as its first President and myself as its first Secretary. The Society

82

still continues its work and has done an enormous amount of good. It has fostered friendly relations between its members and by its scientific meetings, held three or four times a year, it tends to improve the character of the work of the profession in the district. At these meetings papers on medical or surgical subjects are read, cases are described and specimens shown.

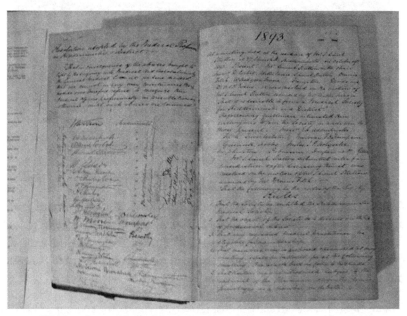

Kidderminster Medical Society – inaugural meeting record – 1893
Courtesy of Kidderminster NHS Treatment Centre

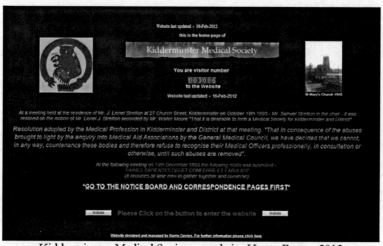

Kidderminster Medical Society – website Home Page – 2012
Courtesy of Kidderminster Medical Society

www.kidderminstermedicalsociety.co.uk

About fifteen years ago the Society instituted the custom of holding an annual summer meeting, to which ladies are invited. These meetings are usually held at some interesting or beautiful place within easy reach by car; papers not strictly medical are read and tea is provided, the whole forming a pleasant summer gathering.

I have been President of the Society for over thirty years and still hold that office. It has often fallen to my lot, as President, to read the paper at the summer meetings, and some of the papers read will find a place in this book.

CHAPTER XI

SOME POINTS IN MEDICAL PRACTICE

Professional secrecy. Cases in Court. Information to employers. Justification of a lie. Precision. A "long time." Consultants and general practitioners. So-called inoperable cases. Heroic operations. Mortality in operations. Persuasion to submit to operation. Interference of outsiders.

The question of professional secrecy often arises. I maintain that any information I obtain from my patients is sacred, and I used to say that nothing on earth would drag it out of me. But I have seen of late that some Judges insist that medical men shall give information in the Courts, and I feel that if I were placed in the position of a witness I should give the required evidence under protest, because I doubt if I could stand the hardship of an imprisonment at my time of life. I think, however, that some young member of the profession should sacrifice himself, and go to prison if necessary, in order to get the law established that we are entitled to withhold information we have obtained from our patients. Lawyers and ministers of religion are privileged to withhold information and it seems to me only just and reasonable that the same privilege should be extended to medical men.

My ordinary method of dealing with inquisitive people is to give them a non-committal answer. If Mrs. J. asks me what is the matter with Mrs. W. I reply, "Oh, nothing very serious." If she questions me further I make another evasion; if she still persists I give her a lesson and ask her how she would like it if people asked about her and I told them what was the matter with her.

I have often been asked by employers to give them information about their workpeople and I have always refused to do so unless the patients have given their permission, and I prefer that this shall be given in

85

writing so that there shall be no mistake. A gentleman who was a very good patient of mine once came to ask me about one of his employees who was suffering at the time from mental disease from which he was never likely to recover, and which was of such a nature that it might have involved the firm in the loss of a great deal of money. Now if I were to give information when the disease is trifling no great harm would be done; but if I did this and an occasion arose when I refused to give any information it would at once be obvious that there was something very wrong; hence the only safe way is always to refuse. I therefore explained to the gentleman in question that I never did give any such information, but that if he wished for a report from me he must first obtain the permission of the patient and his wife and then send me written instructions to report to him. Fortunately he was a sensible man and he did as I suggested. I then reported the condition of the patient to him, thereby saving the firm from a great deal of difficulty.

I have occasionally been placed in such an awkward position that I have been forced into telling a lie rather than reveal the condition of a patient. I unhesitatingly tell the lie and consider myself entirely justified in doing so.

It is very necessary to cultivate the habit of accuracy and precise description. A patient comes in to see me; I say, "Good morning, ma'am; what is the matter with you?" "I don't know, Sir; I came for you to tell me that." Perhaps that is a justifiable rebuke for me. It would have been more accurate if I had asked her what symptoms she was suffering from; if I had, she probably would not have understood me and it would then become my duty to worm all these symptoms out of her. The first question I ask a patient is, "How long have you been ill?" The answer is almost invariably the same, "Oh, a long time." That reply conveys absolutely nothing to my mind. I have often been taxed with untruthfulness when I say this. But surely fifty years might be considered a long time; yet I fancy that if your train came in 20 minutes late on a foggy wintry evening you would feel that you had waited "a long time" on the platform.

I ask a patient how large a certain lump was when he first noticed it. He replies, "It was as large as a nut." He is much surprised when I ask if he means a coconut. Then he says, "A walnut." But even this is not very precise, for some walnuts are three or four times as large as others. The same applies to apples, oranges, eggs, and other things that are sometimes given as a criterion of size. One does not expect the laity, and especially uneducated members of the laity, to give an accurate definition, but a qualified member of the profession may reasonably be expected to do so; yet such vague descriptions have often been given to me by doctors and even today I sometimes see them in the medical press.

Many general practitioners complain that consultants treat them unfairly, and no doubt this is true of some of them. On the other hand, it is quite certain that some general practitioners behave unfairly towards consultants. Here is an instance. Some years ago I was sent for, to see a young lady who was suffering from a surgical complaint. She had been staying in the north of England and her parents had been advised to place her under my care. They lived five or six miles away from the town and I knew that a general practitioner living near them attended the family. I urged them to allow me to invite him to be present when I saw the patient. To this they agreed, and I placed her under his care, acting myself only as consultant. The patient did quite well. Some six months later her father came to me and asked me to take charge of his wife. I explained to him that I could do this only in a consulting capacity. He told me that in spite of my desire to uphold my professional brother they were quite determined not to have him to attend them again. I still told him that I could not attend them, at which he was exceedingly annoyed. I ultimately agreed that I would write to the doctor, and if he agreed to my doing so I would undertake the care of the patient. I wrote to the doctor and explained the position exactly and he replied and thanked me. He wrote that I had acted in accordance with professional etiquette, and that I must certainly not attend the family. The result was that they called in somebody else. I maintain that that doctor behaved very badly. He knew they were not going to have him again in any case, and he acted in this way so that they should not have the man they wanted when they left him.

Exactly the same kind of thing happened in the case of another family attended by the same general practitioner. In both instances I made enemies of the people through acting honourably towards my professional colleague.

Many patients suffering from so-called inoperable conditions may be given a considerable measure of relief, may obtain prolongation of life, and, in isolated instances, even a cure, if we interpret the word 'cure' to mean that the disease never recurs during the lifetime - exceeding ten years - of the patient. It was at one time agreed that if a patient lived for three years after undergoing an operation for malignant disease he was cured. I have never subscribed to that doctrine; I have seen recurrences after much longer periods than three years.

My contention is that many of these sufferers would be far better off if they were dead. Indeed, if they belonged to the lower orders of the animal creation we should be punished for trying to keep them alive; we should have to put an end to them. Therefore, in my opinion, no matter how heroic an operation may be, if there is only a 1 per cent chance of success, I would undertake it, provided always that the patients and their relations thoroughly understood the risks they were running. To perform a dangerous operation and tell the patient and his friends that it is nothing of importance and that there is no danger in it is to my mind criminal. I have performed many such dangerous operations, but I have never done so without explaining the position and the risks and letting the patients decide whether they will have the operation or not.

All operative surgeons have to face a mortality risk. You may perform an operation that has a mortality of only 1 in 500, but you are going to meet with that death if you are dealing with large numbers, as we do. It has often been remarked to me that such fatalities always seem to occur just in those cases where one particularly does not want them to happen. For instance, take such as operation as ventrofixation of the uterus. I had done a large number of these operations without a death when I operated upon an elderly relative of mine, and she died as a result of it. But I do not regard that as the one case where I should not have wanted a death. I never want any of my patients to die; to me it is not a question of relationship, nor is it a question of position or money. I admit, however, that I do not want an imbecile or an idiot to live.

It is often very difficult to persuade patients to undergo an operation, and this difficulty is greatly accentuated if their symptoms are not acute. Many of the patients one has to interview are not well educated and one has to put the position before them in a simple yet forcible way that they can understand. Early in my career I formulated the following as a very suitable method. I say to a patient: "Suppose you are walking down a road and you come to a point where it divides into two. There is a sign-post on the right-hand side on which is written that 'Out of every 100 persons who go down this road 20 will die.' On the left-hand side the sign-post has, 'Out of every 100 persons who go down this road 1 will die.' Which road will you take?"

Then I explain that taking the left-hand road means undergoing the operation. I have found this way of putting it answers very well. To those persons who are more intelligent I have amplified it by saying: "Supposing that you, as a sensible person; decide to go down the road where only 1 out of 100 is going to die, and you should happen to be that one, does it prove that you are unwise? On the other hand, if you go down the road where 30 out of every 100 are going to die, and you happen to be one of the survivors, is that any proof that you are not exceedingly rash?"

Of course there are some intelligent, high-minded persons to whom the need for the operation has to be fully explained. On two memorable occasions I had patients refuse to submit to the operation of colostomy, and I am by no means sure that they were unwise, for the extra period of existence that the operation would have secured would have been a period of misery to them. One of them said to me, "Do you consider it is a duty to my God that I should have this done?" and I unhesitatingly replied in the negative.

Another difficulty that surgeons meet with is the interference of outsiders; they may be relations or friends, or sometimes merely acquaintances. So many people are fond of explaining that they know of a similar case that had been treated successfully in some different way, and they suggest that this should be tried. Sometimes this sort of thing is very troublesome.

CHAPTER XII

GRATITUDE

Definitions of gratitude. Money payment not everything. Gratitude after fatality. Accounts contested. Ingratitude and injustice. Alleged mistakes. Risks to life. A bad debt. Case of delirium tremens. Dishonourable treatment. Saved from ruin. Presents. Self-denial. Preferential payments. Acting as trustee.

'A sense of appreciation of favours received, accompanied with goodwill towards the benefactor; an emotion or sentiment of thankfulness; being thankful, appreciation of and inclination to return kindness'. These are dictionary definitions of gratitude. In my opinion gratitude is the natural response of the heart to kindness intended or received, the impulse, the desire to show a proper appreciation of the favour and to requite it if possible. It is easy to express gratitude, by well-chosen words, sometimes accompanied by gestures and tears. Often those who are the most demonstrative are really the least grateful. To be genuine, gratitude should be accompanied by some practical proof. We should desire to requite the favour done to us, and in doing so we should willingly impose upon ourselves some self-denial.

Some imagine that a money payment to a medical man removes all obligation. Two wealthy women actually told me this. It was no use arguing with them. They could not, or would not, see that no amount of money could pay for some services; they considered the payment of money was all-sufficient. What such people lose! How differently you feel towards a man who sends you a case of wine, a turkey, or a box of cigars on every anniversary of the operation you performed for him, thereby saving his life! Or towards the poor patient who sends a needlework dolly, a few eggs, or a bunch of flowers from a cottage garden! These express quite as much gratitude as the more valuable gifts, and I appreciate them quite as much.

Some services demand more gratitude than others; it may be they merit a life-long continuance of gratitude. Few callings in life have more experience in this subject than the medical profession.

> "God and the doctor both alike adore,
> But only when there's danger, not before,
> The danger o'er, both are alike requited,
> God is forgotten and the doctor slighted."

These are oft-quoted words and unfortunately there is much truth in them. Still, in a long experience I have found some notable exceptions and I have sometimes been cheered by unmistakable evidence of genuine gratitude.

Thanks after an operation are frequent, but if the patient dies we often receive slights, if not reproaches. The relatives leave us, they avoid us and may even cut us. All sorts of unkind things are said about us. Some of these are actionable, but I have always thought it unwise to take any action in such cases. If we win, our opponents are considered martyrs; if we lose, they say it serves us right, and we probably lose our practices, or at least part of them.

People are apt to forget that our work is much heavier and more anxious in cases that terminate fatally. Nevertheless in some few instances this is realised. To be thanked for one's services after a fatality is indeed gratifying and I have experienced this satisfaction several times. In a commercial community, where most things, if not all, are governed and measured by £. s. d., it is quite usual to find that after a protracted illness, involving the medical men in much work, anxiety and loss of rest, sometimes to the extent of injuring his health or even shortening his life, the account for the professional fees is contested. We may have to fight a case in the Court or else accept a smaller sum, combined with insults of varying degree, some going so far as to impute dishonest motives, and the patient probably transfers his patronage to another member of the profession. I regret that truth compels me to state that in many instances the other man is acquainted with the facts and will even in some instances go to the length of quoting a lower fee. Nor is he always particular as to veracity. He will give it out in professional circles that his fees are the highest while at the same time he is accepting nominal payment in order to capture patients.

Patients not only transfer their own patronage, but they use all their powers of persuasion to induce their acquaintances to leave a doctor they have themselves left. Especially is this the case if they have transferred because of the fees. They will not allow anybody to think that they are mean or that they are either unable or unwilling to pay the highest fee for medical attendance. Hence they proclaim incompetence, carelessness, or anything that will injure a man who has perhaps saved their lives or the life of someone dear to them. Then they will extol the virtues and the skill of the man to whom they have transferred, even though they know that their statements are untrue. They do not seem to realise that they are ungrateful and unjust and that their desire to injure their former medical attendant may do serious harm not only to him but also to those dependent upon him; it may even threaten his very existence. I sometimes wonder if they have ever read with understanding Shylock's words: "You take my life when you do take the means whereby I live."

Some patients condemn a doctor who has attended them for years and who has perhaps saved one or more lives in their family, because they imagine that he has made a mistake, an error in diagnosis or treatment. They do not seem to realise that they are thereby constituting themselves judges of intricate professional questions and opinions. Some of them would be surprised to know that a single case submitted to experts might produce several different diagnoses and several different methods of treatment. I am quite aware that some mistakes are justifiable and some are unjustifiable; but I fail to understand how anyone who has not the knowledge possessed by a qualified practitioner can so far delude himself as to imagine that he is capable of deciding which of several different professional opinions is correct.

Suppose a doctor does make a mistake. Surely it is not necessarily criminal. Is he the only man in the world who is never to make one? He would be a marvellous specimen of humanity if he went through life without making a single mistake. What about politicians, clergyman, and financiers? Even the cleverest will make a mistake sometimes. Lawyers will spend days in the trial of a case and after exhausting every means of investigation to discover the truth they may arrive at a wrong decision. All these are forgiven; indeed, it is looked upon more or less as part of the game. But if a doctor fails he at once becomes an enemy to be scouted and insulted until he may have to defend himself in an action at law.

People should never forget past services, and they should realise that no amount of money can repay some services. A body damaged as a result of services rendered to others may cease to live some years earlier than it should do; that is, the mortality rate among medical men is above the average and their expectation of life is worse. Can money pay for the years thus sacrificed? The business man will say, "The more fool he to risk his life for other people!" Yes! But what if this business man is ill and feels that you alone can save him or even hasten his recovery? Then it is, "Ah, doctor! You don't look too well yourself; you ought to get away for a holiday as soon as I am well again." If you remind him that you may have some other patient who desires your attendance, he will say it is absurd to expect you to keep at work always. "Of course you must get away; they must get someone else to look after them!" yet still he insists that you must not go until he is well himself.

Some examples of gratitude, or rather ingratitude, are more flagrant than others, as will be seen by the following concrete cases that have actually occurred to me. I have painted them in colours somewhat different from the reality in order to obscure them, but I have not darkened these colours.

In the early days of my practice I was attending a tradesman who ultimately died, leaving a widow and a young family. I did not know their financial position, but I felt no anxiety about the payment of my fees, which amounted to nearly £50, a sum of great moment to me at that period of my career. My composure appeared to be justified by the fact that the funeral, to which I was invited, was conducted upon a very expensive scale. Imagine my surprise when a few months later I was aroused after midnight to see the widow. On going downstairs I found her with her sister-in-law, in such a state of agitation that she had difficulty in explaining to me that she was in financial trouble. It was the

94

old story. She had got into the hands of a money-lender, and the Sheriff's officer was put into her house to recover £20 plus £5 expenses. She said it would ruin her business if she was sold up. Her brother would lend her half the amount if I would provide the other half. Her sister-in-law confirmed this statement.

I was going away the next morning for a short holiday and I was to pass through the town where the money-lender carried on his business. I saw the man and arranged that he would accept £20 down in full settlement, and I paid it him. On my return home I called upon the widow and asked her to get the £10 her brother had promised. She said he was unable to pay it. In short, I had lost my £20 and also the money due for my professional services. I was so irritated that I went to a celebrated criminal lawyer who practised in the neighbourhood. I told him my story as faithfully as I could. When I had finished he looked at me and smiled. He then said, "I suppose you know she is little better than a prostitute." When I indignantly denied any such knowledge, he replied, "Well, if you don't, I do, and it is generally known. If you bring an action no-one will believe you were such a fool as to lend her £20 and get nothing for it. Go home, write it off as a bad debt, and forget all about it." Very reluctantly I followed his advice. I wonder if she was grateful to me for my attendance and my loan.

A lawyer came in to see me one evening about a client of his who was suffering from a sharp attack of delirium tremens. His people were frightened and anxious to have him removed to safe keeping. I did not care to deal with such cases, but after a great deal of persuasion from the solicitor, who promised to pay all the fees, I agreed to take the patient into my Nursing Home and attend him there; and there he remained until he was discharged cured. The Nursing Home fees were paid and warm expressions of thanks reached me from the patient's wife and the solicitor. Some few months later I met this solicitor and reminded him that he had not sent me my fees. "Oh!" said he, "I am not going to pay you, and my client cannot." On my again reminding him of his promise, he replied, "Yes, but that was only by word of mouth; you have not got it in writing, and I shall deny it." Thereupon I left him and I never spoke to him again. If anyone treats me in a dishonourable manner I avoid any contact with that person in future. I bear him no malice, I would not harm him, nor could I refuse to render him first aid but beyond that I will not go.

I was once attending an elderly man in a serious illness that we feared might end fatally. His wife asked me to find out from him whether he had made a will, and if so, where it was. He told me his will was made and in the possession of a certain solicitor, whom he had appointed as his sole executor. I also discovered that the main part of his estate consisted of real property, the deeds of which were in the safe keeping of the same solicitor. This was the man I had had to deal with in the case just described, and I was so convinced that he was not to be trusted that I persuaded my patient, as soon as he was able, to go to the solicitor's office and demand his deeds. He had some difficulty about this, but he ultimately succeeded in getting possession of them. Within a few months that solicitor had disappeared, leaving a number of people the poorer for his activities. My patient and his wife were overjoyed at their lucky escape. If their deeds had gone the workhouse would have been their sole resource. They were loud in their expressions of gratitude to me. Another lawyer was consulted, another will was prepared, and I was named as executor and trustee, a position I filled for some years, since the old man died soon afterwards. I cannot say I was surprised when I saw the conveyance of another medical man standing outside the house two or three years later. He attended the widow; she smiled at me whenever I saw her and I observed an attitude of indifference. Some ten or fifteen years later the old lady died. I had not communicated with her since she left me and knew of her death only through reading the announcement of it in the newspaper. From her solicitor I learnt that she had made a will and named me as executor. He presumed that I should refuse to act under the circumstances." I replied, "I shall most certainly fulfil my duties," That was the measure of her gratitude to me from saving her from ruin, to say nothing of the professional services I had rendered, which were of such a nature that on occasions they had placed my own life in considerable jeopardy. My feeling towards her was more of pity than resentment, for surely one who can behave in such a way must be devoid of those finer feelings that help to make life worth living and raise us above the level of the lower animals.

People sometimes show their gratitude to their doctor by sending him a present. I have had patients who have sent me more money than I asked for. If I sent an account for £75, they might send me a cheque for £100, and very gratifying it is. Sometimes they give me a picture or a bit of plate. A patient whom we have charged nothing may send us a present. I have no wish to look a gift horse in the mouth, but in some instances where I have done work representing anything up to £300 people who could easily have sent me a gift worth 10 or 20 guineas have sent a thing worth sixpence. It seems to me extraordinary that a man, who writes at Christmas and tells me he can never forget me on this festive occasion, for he knows he owes his life to me, will enclose a sixpenny packet of chocolate. It would be much better to send nothing at all. Some of my most cherished possessions have been trifles given to me by quite poor people out of gratitude, but the kind of thing I have just described looks to me more like ingratitude.

My own idea is that nobody can adequately show gratitude, and nobody really performs an act of charity, unless there is some self-denial in it. It seems to me a great pity that statements should be published in the newspapers to the effect that So-and-so has made a munificent donation, when the amount is altogether inadequate if compared with the value of the estate of the donor. A gift of £5,000 from one person may be less than a halfpenny from another.

Some years ago a man died owing me a considerable sum for professional attendance. I never received anything and I later ascertained that several creditors had been paid in full, so I wrote to the executors for my fees. They told me that they had distributed the estate and there was nothing left for me. They were sons of the deceased and they knew quite well that my fees were due. I was very much annoyed and went to instruct my solicitor to proceed against them. Then to my astonishment I learned that executors have a legal right to make preferential payments to creditors, that is, they can pay any creditors they choose in full and pay the rest nothing. To any ordinary person this seems most unjust. Surely all the creditors should be treated in the same way; but again, "The law's an ass!" I have had to buy all this experience. Why should not somebody else read it in a book?

Members of our profession are often invited to act as trustees. This sometimes lands us in difficulties and teaches us many things. One has to be very careful how one deals with solicitors. If appointed as trustees we can refuse to act; we can put the matter into the hands of the Public Trustee. But my own opinion is that if we are appointed as trustees it is our duty to act, if we possibly can. It is certainly our duty to act if we have promised a patient that we will do so.

CHAPTER XIII

THE POWER OF THE TOP HAT

Victorian. Professional dress. My top hat. Its place at the hospital. Top hat on a "penny-farthing." Bicycle tour. Top hat and scarlet dressing-gown. Unrecognised without top hat. Incident in Dublin.

I have often been reproached or ridiculed for being Victorian, or even what by some people is considered almost an insult, early Victorian. Neither reproach nor ridicule has the slightest effect upon me. Far from being ashamed of being Victorian, or early Victorian, I am rather inclined to glory in it. In my opinion it would be better for us all if more of the Victorian principles, habits, and manners were to be found among us nowadays.

I was brought up and entered upon my practice when frock-coats and top hats were considered almost the hall-mark of professional men. No self-respecting doctor of any standing would have dreamt of appearing in any other garb, at any rate during the exercise of his profession. He would have considered that a lounge suit and a bowler hat would neither earn respect for himself nor show respect for his patients. What he would have thought of the plus-fours and soft caps of the present day I cannot imagine. Times have indeed changed!

Through all the years of my professional life I have remained faithful to my top hat. For more than fifty-five years my top hat was always deposited in a special place by itself in the hall at the hospital, and it was recognised that if anyone wanted to know whether I was in the building or not all that was necessary was to go and see if my hat was in its usual place.

This loyalty to my top hat has led to some amusing incidents. In the early days of my practice one of my brothers dared me to ride, wearing my top hat and frock-coat through the town and up the hill to the hospital on a high bicycle, the so-called penny-farthing. I did it, and a most ridiculous object I must have appeared!

When it was my custom to go for bicycle tours I generally used to start by train and meet my friend at a pre-arranged rendezvous. But on one occasion I was picking up the night train at Wolverhampton and I found it would be more convenient to ride there. My man, who had been with me for several years, was putting my bicycle in order and strapping on the luggage when I came down, dressed in my light knickerbocker suit and a cap. I stood in my yard watching him. He looked round at me two or three times but did not speak. When he had finished adjusting the machine I said to him, "Is it all right now?" He fairly jumped and said, "Why I didn't know you, Sir. I never thought of it being you."

I got on the bicycle and rode out into the street behind my garage. There I met a gentleman riding a bicycle. I had known him for years; he rented an office from me in the next house to mine and I used to see him most days. I wished him Good Evening, and asked him which way he was going. When I found it was the same road as my own I said, "O well then, we can ride together," and we did so for fully two miles until our ways parted. I then wished him Good Night, and went on. I was away on my holiday between a fortnight and three weeks. The day after my return I met this gentleman, and I said to him, "Well, we had a very good holiday." "Oh!" he said, "have you been away for a holiday?" "Yes," I replied, "we got up as far as John o' Groats." "Oh!" he said, "how did you get there?" "Why bicycling of course; how else did you think I should go?" "But you don't ride a bicycle, do you?" said he, "I never heard of your riding a bicycle." "Well," I said, "it's very curious you should say that to me, because you rode with me for the first two miles of my journey." He was quite sure he hadn't. When I explained to him how I had met him in the street, "Good gracious! That wasn't you, was it? I have been worrying my head ever since to find out who that was. I thought it was somebody I ought to know but I could not think who it was." He was a very intelligent man, and was afterwards Mayor of the town, yet he was completely at a loss. I should have thought my voice would have given me away, but it did not.

One night I had an urgent call in the small hours to go at once to see a patient who was bleeding. The distance from my house was between two and three hundred yards. It was beautiful summer weather, and in my anxiety to waste no time I decided to walk down in my dressing-gown. This was bright scarlet in colour, with blue collar and cuffs - a most gorgeous garment that my mother had given me. As I walked through the hall my top hat was in its usual place on the table and quite mechanically I put it on and walked down the town. I did not realise what a ludicrous appearance I must have presented until I found the hat in my patient's hall when I was leaving his house. However, I put it on and walked back home in it.

I was asked by the wife of a doctor, her husband not being available, if I would go and see an urgent accident case. I went and found that an old gentleman of 70 had fallen down and injured his back. He did not appear to know me. I asked him if he had lived in the town all his life, to which he replied "Yes." "And you don't know me?" I asked, rather surprised. "No, Sir, I don't think I have ever seen you before." "I am Mr. Stretton," I said. "Oh! Are you any relation to Lionel Stretton? I knows him all right." "I am Lionel Stretton." "Well now," said he, "I wouldn't have believed it. If you had had your top hat on I should have known you." I fetched my top hat from the hall and put it on, and he knew me at once.

One evening I was attending a public dinner as the guest of a doctor who lived in the neighbourhood. He was late and I spent the time of waiting in conversation with a man I knew quite well. When the doctor arrived he apologised for being late and said to the man with whom I had been talking, "You know Mr. Stretton, of course." "O yes, I know him quite well," was the reply, "but is he here tonight?" I then chimed in: "Yes, I'm here all right." "But," he said, "you are not Mr. Lionel Stretton that's the one I know." "Well, I happen to be Mr. Lionel Stretton." Whereupon he answered, "Then I must apologise, but I've never seen you before without your top hat."

A friend of mine went into a tobacconist's shop in Dublin to buy some cigarettes. He noticed that the tobacconist's one arm did not move quite so freely as the other and, being of an inquisitive disposition, he asked him what was the matter with his arm. "Oh," said the man, "I had that arm shattered in the war and but for a wonderful surgeon who looked after me I should have lost my arm, and perhaps my life too." My friend then wanted to know who the wonderful surgeon was. "Ah!" said the man, "he's a man named Lionel Stretton, of Kidderminster, a wonderful, old gentleman with a white moustache, and he always wears a top hat."

CHAPTER XIV

HUMOURS OF THE PROFESSION

Amusing experiences. A madman. Twins. Beneficial pills. Glass of port. Pipe of tobacco. Tablespoonful of whisky. Bottle of medicine. An original prescription. A stiff ankle. Crow or cackle? Letters. Telegrams. Two carriages for one man. An Irish bull. Two patients, same name. Question of amputation. A lot of vitality. Leg for sale. Cleaning the eyes. A glass eye. Throat examination. Appendix operation. Offer of "long-tails." Legal argument.

The medical profession is rightly regarded as a very serious one; but in the course of our practice we meet with many amusing experiences, and there is no reason why we should not enjoy them ourselves and relate them to others. There are innumerable funny stories about bygone members of the profession, but in this chapter I shall confine myself to amusing experiences of my own or to others of which I have personal knowledge.

A friend and colleague of mine was summoned to examine a young man with a view to certifying him as insane. He rode to the house on his bicycle and propped it against the pavement outside. He entered the room just in time to see the young man jump out of the window, mount his bicycle and ride off on it, gaily shouting ' Ta Ta' as he went.

An old friend of mine, who was surgeon to a Railway Company, was giving evidence on their behalf; it was an action for damages, claimed because a woman who was involved in a railway accident had given premature birth to twins. The opposing Counsel when cross-examining him said, "I understand you are a surgeon." "Yes," "And you practise surgery only?" "Yes." "Then what on earth do you know about twins?" "I have them at home," was my friend's reply.

When my father visited an old lady one day, he said, "Yes, you are decidedly better today. The pill I sent you evidently did you good and I should advise you to take another tonight." The old lady replied, "If you will look in that ornament on the chimney-piece you will find your parcel of pills all sealed up. I thought it would be a pity to deprive somebody else of their benefit."

It is very necessary to be precise in the instructions we give to patients. It is extraordinary how some patients will deliberately take advantage of any indefinite instructions, even though they are fully aware that they are acting contrary to the wishes of their medical attendant. One day when I went to see one of my father's patients the old gentleman said to me: "I have been most obedient to your father's instructions. He told me that I was to have only one glass of port wine a day and I have never taken more since he gave me those orders, but I have had it out of a celery glass." The celery glasses of those days would hold quite a bottle of port wine.

Another man had been advised to limit the quantity of tobacco he was smoking and had promised to be content with one pipe a day. He started off into the town, bought a new pipe, and smoked it every day. About a month later he told me with pride that he had confined himself to one pipe a day, and he showed me the pipe. It was one of those show pipes that are to be seen in tobacconists' windows, and it had a huge bowl that held over an ounce of tobacco.

Another old gentleman, a hunting squire who was getting on in years and rather feeble, was ordered by my father to take a cup of milk with a tablespoonful of whisky in it every morning before he got up. The next morning the butler took him up a tray with a tumbler half full of milk, a silver tablespoon, and a decanter of whisky. "Now, John," said the old gentleman, "Mr. Stretton said that I was to have a tablespoonful of whisky in the milk; hold the tablespoon well over the tumbler and don't mind how much whisky runs over while you are pouring it out."

The directions on medicine bottles are sometimes misread or misunderstood. A gamekeeper was sent by his master to see my father. On his return his master asked him what Mr. Stretton had said to him: "Oh, he told me to be careful in my diet and not take any tea and he thinks I'll soon be right again." "Didn't he give you any medicine?" "O yes, Sir, he gave me a bottle of medicine." "Well, I should like to see it." "Why sure, Sir, I drunk it and I thought it were no use carrying the bottle home, so I throwed him away." Fortunately there was no poison in the medicine or the result might have been very serious.

My father was hurriedly and quite unnecessarily summoned one evening to see an old lady patient. When he had examined her he told her maid to call at his house for a prescription and then take it to his assistant to be dispensed. The prescription was: "Give this troublesome old woman something cheap and nasty." Through some misunderstanding the maid took the note to her mistress, who opened it and read it. The interesting sequel is that my father continued to attend that patient for the rest of her life. She must have had a sense of humour.

During the war a man whose lower extremity I had removed by an amputation through his thigh was sent in due course to an institution where an artificial limb was provided for him. At a later date he was summoned before a Medical Board. When he entered the room he was asked why he walked lame, and he explained that his ankle was stiff. They wrote on his card "Massage and Electrical Treatment." Imagine their surprise when he told them that the ankle was an artificial one.

Some years ago I performed some successful operations upon tendons of the hands and feet, and I prevented the adhesion of the tendons to the skin by covering them with pieces of membrane removed from the inner side of eggshells. Of course the hospital wag told me not to crow over this; but should he not have said cackle?

Letters, telegrams, and telephone messages often cause trouble, but they may have their humorous side. The daughter of a hospital patient once wrote to me: "Dear Sir, Would you be so kind as to let me know what my father died from as I am in a bit of difficulty of having my father's insurance money. Would you let me know if it was a standing disease for years or did it come at once?"

Another patient, a girl whom I had advised to come into hospital for an operation, wrote: "Dear Sir, I will be at your service any time after the 17th of this present month."

One day I got a telegram, "Don't come dead," signed by somebody fifteen or twenty miles away. I wondered if they were expecting me in my coffin. I had not previously been asked to go to the place, but I came to the conclusion that the doctor there had been to see the patient in question and arranged with the family that he should telegraph for me to go and meet him in consultation there, and that the patient had since died. My conclusion was proved correct an hour or so later when I had a telegram from the doctor asking me to go and see this patient with him.

I had sent a wealthy patient abroad for six months. About six weeks later he wrote to his wife that he intended to return earlier. She consulted me and we arranged that I should telegraph to tell him to stay away the full time. As the cost of telegraphing was 8/- a word I made the telegram as short as possible; it read 'Return unwise remain six months.' That appeared to me to be perfectly clear. To my surprise I received a telegram from my patient asking me to explain what I meant. I had to send another telegram containing about five times the number of words in the original one. The patient was a rich man and could well afford to pay for it, but it really did seem to me unnecessary. At a later date when he returned home I had this out with him. He maintained, and said that all his acquaintances in the hotel agreed with him, that my first telegram meant that he was to return home immediately and that it was unwise to remain six months. Had he a right to think that? At any rate it shows how difficult it is to write anything that cannot be misinterpreted.

One snowy winter day I had difficulty in keeping my horse on its legs as I drove up to the hospital in my buggy. I telephoned down to my house to give instructions to have two of my horses roughed. Imagine my surprise when I came out of the hospital to find two of my carriages waiting for me. The coachman declared he had been ordered to bring my Broughams and pair of horses up to the hospital at once. Who made the mistake I did not find out. It was not the 1st April, but the Jehu was an Irishman, and I believe they did play him that trick once. He was a comical fellow. If I asked him in the morning whether it was going to rain his reply always was, "I don't think not, Sir." What he meant I don't know.

Only a year or so ago I ordered some vaccine and arranged that it was to be sent by a certain train, which would be met at the station. It did not arrive. When explaining my annoyance to a member of our medical staff at the hospital - an Irishman - I told him how annoying it was that I had met the vaccine and it did not come; he at once reminded me that I was not an Irishman.

One day many years ago I arrived home to find an urgent telephone message to tell me to go and see a patient I was attending. There was a later message, left personally, to say the patient was so much better that I need not go. I did not go. In the evening an angry husband came to abuse me for not going to see his wife. That was because the two patients happened to have the same name.

Patients and their relatives often make amusing remarks. I once told a woman that her husband's leg was in a bad condition and that if it did not improve we should have to discuss the question of amputation; to which she replied, "We have already tried that, Doctor."

A clergyman told me that he had asked the daughter of one of his parishioners what was the matter with her mother, to which she replied, "Mr. Stretton has not told us exactly, but he says as 'ow she had a lot of vitality and I expect that is very serious."

Some patients have quaint ideas. A man was brought to the hospital with gangrene of the leg and there was nothing for it but to amputate the limb to save his life. Although I did my best for him he not only withheld any sign of gratitude but he tried in an ingenious way to invert the obligation. In the weary hours of the night he called the Nurse to his bedside and said to her, "What do you think Mr. Stretton would give me for my leg that he cut off?" Such an example of callous ingratitude can best be met by a smile.

On several occasions I have been told by patients that I had removed their eyes, cleaned them and put them back again, when as a matter of fact I had only slit up their canaliculi.

Some years ago I removed an eye from a man sent from the Workhouse Infirmary into the Hospital, and I was instructed by the Master of the Workhouse to get an artificial eye for him. I asked what quality they wanted. "Oh," he said, "we must have one of the best - one that he can see well with." He ought to have known better.

One day I was examining a child that was supposed to have large tonsils. The child was being held on the nurse's knee and I was kneeling on a hassock trying with the help of a spoon to look into her throat. Suddenly the mother rushed at me and hit me such a violent blow on the side of my head that it sent me sprawling onto the floor. Fortunately I was able to look at the humorous side of the somewhat undignified situation, but at a later date when I removed the child's tonsils I took particular care that the mother was kept out of the way.

One day a Ward Sister at the hospital came to me and said that one of the men patients had refused to have his appendix out. "I'll go and talk to him," I said, and I went and talked to him. When I had finished he looked up at the Sister and said, "Could anybody refuse him, Sister?" Within a quarter of an hour his appendix was out and he was back in bed, and he has lived to thank me on several occasions since.

Some years ago an old poacher whom I had been attending came to see me one day and told me he had had a lucky haul. He had about a dozen "long-tails" (pheasants). Would I like four or five of them at 1/- each? He said the Vicar had had four. I told him that the Vicar might like to have them, but I would rather not. Possibly he invented the story of the Vicar in the hope that it might induce me to have some of his "long-tails."

Patients often tell me funny stories. One man told me about a legal argument between Peter and the devil. They could not agree and the devil said he would obtain legal advice on the point in question. After obtaining this advice he came and told Peter that the law was on his side. Peter at once said he must give in; he was unable to contradict him because he had got no lawyers up in his place whom he could consult.

CHAPTER XV

MISTAKES OF THE PROFESSION

Scope of chapter. Varieties of mistakes. A case of faith-healing. Sarcoma of knee-joint. Gall-stones. Tumour or pregnancy? Cases of malignant disease. Positive opinions. Death under anaesthetic. Prejudice in diagnosis. No advice without examination. Empyema. Over-active surgical interference. The contrary. Concurrent disease. Thorough examination. New diseases. Wrong consultants. Wrong medicines. Carelessness. Incorrect death certificate. Amputation of sound finger. Faulty teaching. Morphia as mask. Thoroughness. Charity.

The foundation of this chapter is a paper I read before the Kidderminster Medical Society many years ago. I have shortened it very considerably and yet made additions as the fruit of my later experience.

Mistakes have always been made; they are made at the present time, and I am afraid they always will be made. They are by no means confined to our profession, but their consequences are seldom so serious in other walks of life. It therefore behoves us to be more cautious than the average run of men and to lose no opportunity of fortifying ourselves so far as possible against the perpetration of errors.

It would be outside the scope of this book to make an extensive survey of the mistakes of the profession or to enter very deeply into the causes and character of the mistakes made. This chapter will merely present some general remarks on the subject, include some instances of actual error, and offer certain suggestions as to how some kinds of mistakes may be avoided.

We are all liable to make mistakes. At the outset I will admit that I have made many, and I am certain that nothing is more instructive than a study of our mistakes. Some mistakes are unpardonable, others are pardonable, and some may even have a humorous side. In the last-named category may be included the following story of a mistake of my own; it was made many years ago when I was still in partnership with my father.

I was sent for to see an elderly gentleman - an intimate friend of my family - in consultation with a doctor who was attending him in another town. We agreed that an operation was the only chance of saving his life; but though he realised the seriousness of his condition he refused operation, and his wife supported him in this refusal. He was prepared to die and he gave us his final instructions. He told me he had one great desire; he wished to see my father before he died. At that time my father was away on holiday. I sent him a telegram and he came up at once, arriving home late at night. It was before the days of motor-cars, and in order to see the patient he had to drive nearly twenty miles in his Brougham. I told him I was doubtful whether he would find the old gentleman alive. I was very much pressed with work at the time, but we were on such intimate terms with the family that it fell to my lot to make all the necessary arrangements for the old gentleman, and I was so convinced that he would die that I even went so far as to order his coffin. My father found him alive, laughed and joked with him and cheered him up. He told him that he would give him a bottle of medicine that would cure him. He had the chemist got up in the middle of the night to make up this medicine; the old gentleman took it and was cured, and he lived for ten years afterwards. That was a case of faith-healing. I do not believe the medicine had anything to do with the cure, except for its mental effect. But I do think it possible that a miracle may have happened in his inside, as I know it has happened in other cases, for instance, when Nature has performed a gastro-enterostomy operation on a patient.

The first major operation I performed in Kidderminster, only a few days after I had joined my father in partnership, was an amputation of a limb to remove a sarcoma in the knee-joint of a young man. He had been attending at St. Bartholomew's Hospital for several weeks; they had painted his swollen knee with iodine and told him it would soon be all right again. He said he had seen me at St. Bartholomew's; fortunately for my reputation I had not seen him there. The amputation was quite successful and it prolonged his life.

110

In my early experience of gall-stone surgery - I should rather describe it as my want of experience - I opened an abdomen, found a malignant liver and closed it up again. I was mortified at a later date to learn that another surgeon had removed several stones, thereby effecting the complete relief of the patient's symptoms. Such mistakes are not so likely to occur at the present day, but I would advise any young surgeon who is going to undertake such an operation for the first time that he would be wise to secure the advice and help of an experienced colleague.

An unmarried woman about forty years of age, with an uninviting appearance and unblemished character, came to consult me about an abdominal tumour, which she wished me to remove by operation. I examined her, as I thought, most thoroughly, and eliminated to my satisfaction the possibility of pregnancy. Indeed I almost blamed myself for entertaining even the slightest suspicion against such a highly respectable person. She was admitted to hospital and prepared for operation for the removal of the tumour. Two hours before that operation was to be performed she brought forth a four-month's dead foetus, and she afterwards declared that she was quite unable to account for its presence inside her. I had been on the brink of a precipice and had narrowly escaped having to read a paragraph of the kind that sometimes appears in the lay press under some such heading as "Twins or Tumours at the Hospital?"

An old gentleman under the care of my father was believed by him to be suffering from cancer of the pancreas. I did not agree with this diagnosis and felt satisfied when two eminent members of the profession confirmed my view that there was no organic disease. I felt less satisfied some months later when a portion of the hardened head of the pancreas removed at the post-mortem examination was proved by microscopic examination to be carcinoma.

Positive opinions lead us into many awkward situations and I am afraid that the higher the position we attain the more positive our opinions become; hence it is that many eminent men are led into error.

A lady in a high social position had been seen by three eminent members of the profession in London. She imagined she had a growth in her inside, but they all denied this and pronounced her a neurotic. My father afterwards diagnosed malignant disease and on her death six months later the correctness of his diagnosis was established.

I was called out into the country one night to see a patient who was suffering from strangulated hernia. He was most anxious to avoid operation and after using all my persuasive powers I said, "If you are not operated upon you will certainly die, whereas if the operation is performed immediately I will guarantee that you are cured." He consented to the operation and died before I commenced it - killed by the anaesthetic. My mistake was to guarantee a cure. It was no pleasant duty to inform his son of this tragic occurrence.

It is exceedingly difficult to eliminate prejudice in giving an opinion and I am sure our minds are often biased by a desire to put a good complexion on the case of a friend, especially if he is a member of our own profession. A quondam friend of mine, an eminent young surgeon lately appointed on the staff of his hospital, had symptoms that led him to believe that he was suffering from malignant disease of the intestine. He was seen by several of his colleagues, who all declared that his fears were groundless; yet when he died, as the result of an overdose of morphia, the post-mortem examination proved that his suspicions were correct.

Another form of prejudice is to make up our minds what we are going to see or feel before we see or feel it. A girl was supposed to have swallowed her false teeth, which had got impacted in her oesophagus. She was admitted to hospital and examined by means of the fluorescent screen, when several of those present distinctly saw the plate. But before she was operated upon her mother arrived to tell them that she had found her daughter's teeth in one of her dress pockets at home. If the gentlemen who saw the plate in the oesophagus had not allowed their minds to be prejudiced they would probably have avoided this error.

It is not at all uncommon for friends or relations to ask for our advice casually, but it is unwise to give it without making a routine examination. Clinical mistakes, as Sir W. Jenner said, are more often due to neglect of examination than to lack of knowledge.

Empyema is a condition that is often overlooked and it should ever be remembered as a possible complication of other diseases. Its symptoms may be so masked as to be unrecognised and it behoves a wise House-Surgeon never to discharge a patient from his wards without making an examination of the chest. As I was going round the wards of the hospital one morning the House-Surgeon mentioned to me that one of my patients, who had been suffering from a large gluteal abscess, was going home that day. Something in the look of the patient made me suspicious and I insisted on examining his chest, with the result that I removed several pints of pus from both his pleural cavities and thereby probably saved his life, and perhaps a public scandal.

Some mistakes are the result of too active surgical interference; for instance, one of the leading surgeons in London told me how he had once wounded the brachial artery when performing the old-time operation of bleeding.

On the other hand, if our action is insufficient we may meet with equally disconcerting results. Who has not witnessed the loss of a finger as the result of a whitlow? In reviewing such a case we generally find that the incision was too long delayed and, when undertaken, ended in a small superficial puncture instead of a bold deep incision. This is an example of the dictum "Spare the knife and spoil the finger."

Failure to realise the presence of a concurrent affection is another source of error. There is no greater tragedy than the finding of a corpse in a police cell when the prisoner has been detained for supposed drunkenness. But even if our diagnosis of drunkenness is absolutely correct we should figure very badly in the morning paper if we had not ascertained that the prisoner was suffering from a fracture which, owing to our failure, had become complicated.

I admit that it is very difficult always to avoid this form of error. In the majority of cases it is possible, and in such cases it is right to make a thorough examination, but in some cases it would be highly improper to look for what can only be an occasional occurrence. Such examples are particularly to be found when operating upon the abdomen. If sufficient is found to account for the symptoms I do not think we are justified in making a thorough examination of all the contents of the abdomen, and if the patient is in a bad condition it would be absolutely wrong to do so.

The mistakes due to insufficient examination are, however, frequent. Only quite recently I heard of a case in which a surgeon had removed a stone from the bladder and left two behind. No doubt he felt satisfied at the result of his operation, but he should have had in his mind the possibility of more stones being there. In the year 1924 I removed 52 stones from a bladder.

There is one form of error that occurs through the fact that the medical attendant is totally ignorant of the condition. Take, for instance, anthrax. This disease is seen by only a very small percentage of the profession, and those who have not seen it are hardly likely to take enough interest in the matter to be able to suspect it even when brought in contact with a case. Where should most of us be with a case of sleeping sickness or bubonic plague? I confess that I should be quite unable to diagnose either of these conditions; but I cannot help feeling that we ought to recognise the fact when we come in contact with a disease new to us, and then we ought immediately to ask for an opinion that will help us in arriving at a true interpretation of the symptoms.

As an example of the multitude of matters we ought to be informed about I may mention the possibility of recommending the wrong consultant. We often prescribe the wrong medicines and we ought always to bear in mind that some of our drugs are poisons and some of those poisons have a cumulative effect. Only recently I saw a case of peripheral neuritis due to the continuous use of a prescription containing arsenic.

Errors due to carelessness are unpardonable. Such are the giving of lotions, liniments, or other poisons instead of medicines, errors in compounding and prescribing, etc.

Under the category of carelessness comes the case of the man who signed a death certificate of acute pneumonia for a patient he had been attending for an illness due to a fall from a loft. The post-mortem examination showed a fracture 7 inches long at the base of the skull,

114

extending from a wound at the back of the head, while the lungs were perfectly normal.

Two young surgeons amputated a boy's finger. They gave an anaesthetic and performed a bloodless operation. They were well pleased with their afternoon's work, but not so pleased the next morning when the irate father of the patient told them that they had removed a sound finger instead of the diseased one. They escaped lightly with a payment of £15 compensation. The boy bought a bicycle with the money, and I removed the diseased finger gratuitously at the hospital.

Faulty teaching is sometimes given in lectures. For instance, students are advised to give morphia for the relief of pain. I know that some surgeons adopt this practice, but I maintain that it is wrong. If a dose of morphia is given it masks all the symptoms, and we may fail to recognise the early symptoms of haemorrhage, peritonitis, or perforation, and so lose the opportunity of rendering the immediate surgical aid that would save a life.

I would put in a plea for more thoroughness. Whenever I find myself in error I advise myself to make a more thorough examination in the future. There can be no greater attribute to a surgeon than thoroughness and nothing will better enable him to avoid mistakes.

Finally, while putting ourselves under discipline we ought to use Christian charity in judging the mistakes of others, remembering always that "To err is human, to forgive is divine."

CHAPTER XVI

SOME ALARMING EXPERIENCES

Experiences with patients and when travelling. Delirium tremens. A loaded revolver. Another loaded revolver. Anaesthetic. Stranded in Germany. Inefficient chauffeur. Motor accident. Wind-storm.

In 1934 I read a paper at the summer meeting of the Kidderminster Medical Society on some alarming experiences of my professional life, and that forms the basis of this chapter. Some of the alarming experiences have been connected with the patients themselves, others with travelling to see them; of these latter experiences some have already been described in the chapter on conveyances. Some of the experiences have a humorous side, but that is generally not appreciated until later.

I was sent for one evening to a house on the outskirts of the town to see a confirmed drunkard who was subject to violent attacks of delirium tremens. When I arrived at the house I found a crowd of people outside, including the man's wife, whom he had turned out into the street, some relatives and neighbours and a stalwart policeman. They told me the man in the house was mad; they had heard him smashing up the crockery and furniture. I naturally thought the policeman would go in to see what was happening, but no! I had to go in first and he followed me. When we got into the kitchen the floor was like a shingle beach, with broken crockery all over it. The drunkard was an enormously strong fellow who could easily have crushed the life out of me. Fortunately he knew me and was quite docile when I spoke to him, but he had to be put under restraint. In justice to the police I ought to add that I understand they have no right to enter a man's house.

On another occasion I was summoned in the middle of the night to a house outside the town. When I arrived I found the drive gate locked,

117

but I could see some figures moving about in the shrubbery and soon the wife came to me. She asked me if I would mind getting over the gate, because her husband had locked it and had the key. I got over the gate and then she told me that her husband was mad with drink; he had turned them all out of the house and was in there alone with a loaded revolver. "Do you expect me to go in to him?" I asked. "O yes," she said, "he won't hurt you; he will be quite quiet when he sees you." I was younger in those days or perhaps I was more courageous, though I do not think I ever possessed more than the average share of courage. However, I walked into the house, and there was the man with his revolver. I asked him to put the horrid thing down and fortunately he did so, though he might just as easily have shot me. It was not a very pleasant experience and I have often wondered since if it was fair to my wife and family to have taken such a risk.

These two men were moderate drinkers in comparison with another man, who belonged to my own profession and had been a life-long friend of mine. He almost worshipped the ground I trod on and I had had many talks with him about his intemperate habits, not only intemperance in drink but in other things too. I believe on one occasion he ate sixteen poached eggs on ham for his tea, and he would think nothing of drinking two or three bottles of whisky in an evening. One morning I was summoned to go and see him. When I arrived I was shown up into his bedroom. Nobody dared go near him except an old midwifery nurse he was very fond of. When I walked into the room he was standing in front of the fire. He was an enormous man over 6 feet in height; he weighed 20 stone and was so strong that it would have been futile for me to attempt to struggle with him. The nurse sidled up to me and whispered, "Beware of the pistol!" Before I could take any action my friend levelled his revolver at my head and said with a scowl and a variety of expletives, "I'm not going to listen to any of your cant and if you start lecturing me I'll blow your brains out." It was an uncomfortable situation but I instantly decided on my course of action. There was a large bottle of gin on the table. I said to him, "I have not come here to talk cant or to lecture you in any way whatever. What's that you are drinking?" "It's gin." "Well," I said, "have some by all means," and I poured him out a tumblerful of it, which he drank off as if it had been water. I then invited him to smoke a cigarette with me; he sat down and we both smoked and chatted about old times. I stayed with him for about half an hour; all the time he kept a tight hold of his revolver and I was wondering how best to get away from him. Would it be wise to walk out naturally and risk having a bullet in my back, or would it be safer to walk out backwards so that I could try to dodge a shot if it came? I decided it would be better to walk quietly out of the room as if nothing had happened, so I wished him Good Morning, and walked out. At each step I took I felt that I might have a bullet in me; but I escaped unhurt, though when I got downstairs I felt considerably older than when I went up. If he had shot me his remorse would have been very great; yet he went on drinking until it killed him.

Alarm is not always evident at the time. Some years ago I was administering an anaesthetic to a robust young man at the dentist's. He became so violent that even five of us had difficulty in restraining him. Eventually I got him well under the anaesthetic. Some days later I learnt that when the man came round they found a loaded revolver in his pocket. No doubt he had been trying to get at it when he was struggling with us. It was a good lesson, but we could hardly insist upon searching a man's pockets before administering an anaesthetic.

I had a rather alarming experience when I was travelling on the Continent in 1889, though it certainly had a humorous side. We had come up the Rhine by boat from Cologne to Bingen, where we were to take the train for Heidelberg. When we were getting into the carriage on the train one of the officials came and ordered us forward into a carriage much nearer the engine. In this carriage, as usually happens, a German - an analytical chemist - was very anxious to practise his English on me. While we were talking there was a sudden jolt and on looking out of the window we saw that the last carriage had become detached from the train and rolled down the embankment. The train was stopped; there was no end of excitement and the injured passengers were brought up out of the coach that had rolled over - the very one we should have been in if we had not moved forward. I said to the German who had been talking to me that I supposed it was my duty to let them know that I was a surgeon. I was immediately pressed into service and while I was looking after the injured passengers the train with my friends in it went on without me.

There was I, separated from my party, unable to speak German, stranded with a lot of Germans who could not talk my language, and with no money and no tickets, for they had all gone on in the train. Fortunately I had a pipe and some tobacco, and ultimately a train came along and carried me on to Mannheim. There a crowd of excited officials gathered round me, eager to get particulars of the accident from me; finding they could not make much headway they fetched a smiling young lady to act as interpreter. When I had given them the information they wanted she told me I should have to go about two miles to another station. Would I like to go in some conveyance? As I had no money I chose to walk. A youth was sent with me and he talked the whole time; it might have been interesting if I could have understood what he said. When I reached the other station I found about half a dozen platforms from which trains were constantly departing. As every train went out I had to go and shout out Heidelberg. Eventually I was nodded at and I got into the right train and reached my destination about midnight. My friends met me at the station; they had been telegraphing all up the line to find out what had become of me.

I have had several alarming motoring experiences. One of the most inefficient chauffeurs I was obliged to employ during the War was a very timid driver and his limit of speed was 15 miles an hour. But he went round blind corners at the same rate and to my mind he was the most dangerous chauffeur I ever had. Once when he came round a blind right-angled corner at 15 miles an hour he found a trap coming in the opposite direction. He could not get out of the way, and the shaft of the trap went through the back of the seat that he was sitting upon.

One evening when my own chauffeur was driving me there were some children running along the grass on our nearside and I saw that the foremost child had taken no notice of our coming. I said to my man, "Look out! That child is deaf. Go very slowly." The child suddenly turned round, saw our headlights and rushed straight at them just as a moth will fly into a flame. Of course the car went over her, but we were going so slowly that the man was able to pull up when we had got about half the length of the car over her body. I got out of the car thinking she was probably killed. However, before we could do anything she crawled out from under the car, and except for a lacerated wound on her forehead she seemed none the worse. I took her home and dressed the

120

wound. I intended looking after her until she had completely recovered, but her father was so abusive that I simply gave him my card and left them. I never heard any more about it.

One danger to which we are exposed is a wind-storm. I had an experience of a very violent one some years ago. I had to start out in my carriage one Sunday morning. When I had got about a mile and a half out of the town I found two chimneys blown down off the first house I visited; at the next house the windmill was blown down and wrecked. I went a couple of miles farther and all the way parts of branches of trees were flying about. The next house where I called had a flag-staff in front of it; that was blown down with a great crash while I was there. There was a short drive up to the next house I went to, and while I was there two trees were blown down across the drive and we had to get out through a field. During the next call I made two elm trees were blown down while I was in the house and one of them had to be cut through before we could get away. In one place on the way home there was a large tree blown down across the road and we had to go home another way. The street on the way to my stables was covered with tiles end slates that had been blown off the roofs, and when I got into my stable-yard I found that a wall about 12 to 14 yards long and 8 feet high was lying flat on the ground. We were very lucky to reach home without an accident.

CHAPTER XVII

SOME LEGAL EXPERIENCES

Fear of Court. Death under anaesthetic. Dental operation. Uncertainty of law. Inheritance of fortune. Gratitude. Gain and loss. Statute of Limitations. Expert evidence. Relative terms in Court.

I have had many legal experiences and the greater part of this chapter is taken from an address I gave to the Kidderminster Medical Society on this subject in 1927.

It is curious how some people will bluster and fight and refuse to listen to any compromise; yet when it comes to the final round they will collapse rather than face any legal proceedings. I had an instance of this when I was once unfortunate enough to be dragged into a quarrel between two medical men. I made every effort at reconciliation, and when this failed I suggested arbitration, which was also refused. The one man continued to write abusive postcards to the other, generally ending them with "Now bring your action." He assured me that he had ample justification and said he was most anxious to take the case into Court, but he refused to tell me anything or accept my advice. His opponent assured me that he was not vindictive, that he did not desire heavy damages, but merely a nominal amount, to be paid to the hospital, and an order that the annoyance should cease. Eventually a writ was issued and immediately after this the offender was begging for mercy and trying to get the best terms he could. I believe he had to pay about £200 and costs, a small part of which was handed to the hospital. Memories can be very short!

When hospitals enter into any law case we always find that some men will try to excuse them, while others seem only too anxious to blame them.

I recently read an account of a case in which a patient was killed in a hospital through the administration in error of carbonic acid gas instead of oxygen. At the inquest the anaesthetist explained that the cylinders of carbonic acid gas had a green band painted vertically on each side half-way up from the bottom. He thought the cylinders should be painted green all the way up so that there could be no mistake. The coroner gave a verdict of death by misadventure and stated that there was no evidence of negligence on the part of the anaesthetist or the hospital. It seems to me that if the anaesthetist knew that the green bands went only half-way up he should have exercised more care in examining them, and if he thought the cylinders should be painted green all over he should have asked for this to be done before he killed anyone.

Some years ago I read an account of the case of a girl who died after swallowing a piece of tooth. Her mother sued a dental surgeon, alleging negligence in connection with the attempted extraction of a tooth at a dental hospital. It was stated that the crown of the tooth broke during the operation. The girl suffered from pneumonia after the extraction and during the illness she coughed up a piece of tooth. The jury returned a verdict for the mother and she was awarded £150 damages. The foreman stated that on the evidence before them the jury thought that the general committee and the management committee of the hospital were deserving of censure; they considered there should have been a tighter hold on the management and the officers of the hospital. How the committee could be held deserving of censure passes my comprehension, nor can I imagine any regulations they could draw up that would prevent such a catastrophe.

Barristers have several times warned me that law is uncertain. On one occasion I said to an eminent barrister, "You cannot possibly lose this case." He agreed with me, but he lost the case. He took it to the Court of Appeal and lost again; then he took it to the House of Lords, where he was finally beaten. The case was one that is often quoted in connection with the Workmen's Compensation Act. It was an action by a widow claiming compensation for the loss of her husband, who died of anthrax. At the time it was tried anthrax was not a scheduled disease. In my evidence I explained the three varieties of anthrax. In the case in question the infection was through the conjunctiva, and the barrister agreed with me that in order to establish a claim for an accident the

124

plaintiff must prove that there was an abrasion of the conjunctiva caused at his work. The Judge's decision was to the effect that an accident implied the use of force, and even if the force was so slight as the blowing of a germ on to the conjunctiva it was an accident and the widow was entitled to the compensation. Another Judge might have given a different verdict, but this decision was upheld and the widow was paid the compensation.

Some law cases have a humorous side, but they may be very costly and it is usually wise to avoid going to law if possible. But however we may try to avoid law we are at times forced into it, especially if we possess a strong sense of justice. This sense of justice has several times impelled me to take action, with interesting results. Here is an instance. Many years ago I knew an elderly spinster whose only brother possessed nearly £20,000. When he died he left his sister £100 a year, and the residue of his estate to his daughter, his wife having predeceased him. Soon after his death some kindly disposed person told his daughter that she was illegitimate; it was supposed that this caused her to go wrong, for she eloped with a married man. They set sail for Australia, and before starting the girl made a will leaving all she possessed to the man. On the way to Australia they were shipwrecked and drowned. The lawyer in charge of the estate informed the deceased man's sister that she could have no claim to the money - though she was his nearest living relative for two reasons: (1) the girl was illegitimate and therefore if she had willed it to anyone who had predeceased her the money belonged to the Crown; (2) if two individuals of different sex are drowned in a shipwreck and there is no evidence to show which of them died first the law assumes that the male is the survivor.

I asked the lady if she was going to accept this opinion that she had no claim to the money, or if she intended to put up a fight for herself. She told me she had no money to fight the case. Knowing that she had some wealthy cousins, I recommended her to ask them for help, which she did; it was refused. That was when I came in. I instructed my solicitor to act for her, though I knew that if we lost I might have to pay £500 in costs. It was a long and wearisome business, for the case occupied nearly two years. First, we had to get the registers of many churches searched - a task ultimately crowned with success; the entry of the marriage of the lady's brother was discovered and his daughter

125

proved to be legitimate. That put the claim of the Crown out. Next, we ascertained that a survivor from the wreck was living in Sydney, Australia, and we were able to get an affidavit from him stating that he saw the man and woman clinging to a spar, when a wave came and washed them under. After a few moments he saw the woman come to the surface, but not the man. That put the claim of the man's widow out, with the result that we won our case. The elderly spinster came into the whole of the money, which enabled her to live in great comfort for about twenty years.

The sequel to this case is interesting, though perhaps the lawyer ought not to have told it me. The good lady made a will, and she left the greater part of her fortune to the cousins who had refused to help her to establish her claim to it. She left me £100 in recognition of my help and the risk I had run; but this legacy was cancelled in a later will when her gratitude had still further evaporated. Nevertheless she made me her executor, which gave me the trouble of arranging her funeral and settling up her estate. Some might say I was foolish to take the responsibility of this case, but I did it from a sense of justice and I expect I should do the same again in similar circumstances.

If you go to law you may win your case and lose your money, which is not very satisfactory. I have had several experiences of this. In one instance the sum involved was £200. I was told by my barrister that if I fought and won, the case would be taken to the House of Lords. Assuming that I won right through, it would cost me about £2,000; if I lost, it would cost me £10,000. I let it go.

There are points of law that we learn by experience and the following is an example of a point with which most of the general public are not acquainted. A relative of mine, a man of independent means and supposed to be comfortably off, often told me how fortunate he was in having a solicitor who looked after his interests so well and yet never charged for his services. I had my doubts about that solicitor and I urged my relative to allow me to look into his affairs, particularly on one occasion when he asked me to be surety for him for an overdraft at the bank. When he died I found that all his property was mortgaged to the said solicitor, the interest charged was 1 or 2 per cent more than the usual rate, and no allowance had ever been made for income tax, which

126

is usual in such transactions. My relative was dead, and the only satisfaction I could get was an assurance from the solicitor that he had agreed to forgo the income tax - an assurance I did not believe.

I eventually bought up the remnant of the estate; out of a £25,000 estate only about £2,000 was left. Then the solicitor suddenly sprang upon me an account for professional services to my late relative; it amounted to over £600 and covered a period of 25 years. "Well," I said to my own solicitor, "we need not pay that. We can plead the Statute of Limitations," which means that you are not liable to pay any account more than five years old. However, we asked for particulars, and they came in reams: "To interview with Mr. -- 6/8; To sending telegram to Mr. -- 3/4, cost of telegram 1/6." There were all sorts of such details, 25 years old, and it was impossible to check them; the account had never been delivered. Now comes in the curious fact that astonished me so much. A solicitor is not subject to the Statute of Limitations, that is to say, he can recover fees, no matter how longstanding they may be, so long as he has in his possession any deeds belonging to his client. That seems to me a most iniquitous thing. This should teach people never to allow their solicitor to retain their deeds in his office; the proper place for them is the bank. I wanted to fight this man to show him up, but unfortunately at that period of my career I was not well enough off to do this, or he would certainly have had to go through the Court.

From a professional point of view some of the most interesting legal cases are those in which we are asked to give expert evidence. It is true that we do not run any financial risk, but it is generally found that in such cases the medical witnesses on one side will swear black, while those on the other side, with equal vehemence, will swear white. I do not suggest that their evidence is deliberately untrue, although a certain judge is said to have described three grades of lying witnesses: (1) the liar, (2) the damned liar, and (3) the expert witness. I think it is possible that these witnesses regard the case from different aspects, and they are unconsciously prejudiced in forming their opinions. To my mind this is a very black page in the history of a noble profession.

I was once giving evidence in the Court in a workman's compensation case; it was of more than ordinary importance and the Insurance Company concerned, wishing to evade the payment of compensation, had brought down a barrister of some note from London. I was there as the consulting surgeon in the case. The ordinary medical attendant gave the surgical evidence in chief and, owing to his inexperience and consequent inability to give evidence properly, he had a most uncomfortable time in the box while under cross-examination by the London barrister. When I was cross-examined the Barrister said:

"I suppose you agree with the serious nature of the injury, as described by the previous witness?" "I do."

"And you heard the evidence of the deceased bricklayer's labourer that the injury was caused by a slight tap from a fragment that he had chipped off a brick?" "I did."

"Now can you believe that a slight tap from a fragment of brick could cause the serious injuries that have been described?"

"I am afraid I do not understand your question."

"What? Don't you understand the English language?"

"I hope I do."

"Then what cannot you understand about my question?"

"I do not understand what you mean by 'a slight tap'".

"Oh, I see. I ought to have brought a dictionary here for you. Do you understand what I mean by a severe blow?"

"No! 'A slight tap' and 'a severe blow' are relative terms and they convey absolutely nothing to my mind."

The Judge. "The doctor is quite right. I think you had better not pursue the question any further."

That barrister lost his case and the compensation was awarded. A circumstance of this nature often has a great effect in deciding cases in the Court.

An interesting sequel to this was provided by a friend to whom I told the story. He said to me, "But of course you know what 'a slight tap' means." "No," I said, "I don't. Can you tell me?" "Yes," he said, as he touched the back of his hand with his finger, "that is 'a slight tap.'" "Well," I said, "that is very interesting to me. Last week a man came into my consulting room at the hospital with a black eye. It was so swollen that he could not open his eyelids on that side. I asked him how it had happened and he replied, "A pal of mine gave me a slight tap on the eye." Which of these men was correct?

130

CHAPTER XVIII

CHURCH STREET SUPPER AND BRECKNELL'S CHARITY

Midsummer Eve Custom. Peace and Good Neighbourhood. Origin of Supper.
"Maiden Woman." John Brecknell. Minute book. Hosts. J.G. Brecknell as guest.
Report, 1924. Speech, 1925. "Difference." "Subsist." Brecknell bequest. Tombstone.
Gratitude. Friendly intercourse. Peace.

A curious old custom is still observed in Church Street, Kidderminster, when every Midsummer Eve, June 23rd, a supper is held to which the male inhabitants of the street are invited and at which the time-honoured toast of "Peace and Good Neighbourhood" is drunk. When Midsummer Eve falls on a Sunday the supper is held on Saturday, June 22nd. The following account of the origin of the supper is copied from the minute book of the meetings and is the first entry in the book:-

> "Tradition informs us that a Maiden Woman left to the inhabitants of the Church Street in Kidderminster the sum of Forty Shillings to be put out to Interest and that the Person in whose hands the said sum was Entrusted should engage to provide as many farthing loaves as the Interest would pay for, in order to give One to every Child that was either born or lived in the Church Street, and should also engage to invite to his House upon Midsummer Eve every Male Inhabitant of the said Street to see to the faithful distribution of the said loaves.

> "Tradition also says, that many Years ago, the said Forty Shillings was lost by being lent to some poor Person inhabiting a House up an Entry behind the front of the Church Street, but the Original Sum was again made up by some well disposed People. And it was then agreed that no Person who did not Inhabit a House to the front of the said Street should ever have it again, nor

any other person but such as the majority of the Inhabitants assembled should approve and who should provide two Surety's to engage with him for the repayment of the said money with interest.

"It seems to be the principal intention of the original Donor, that the Male Inhabitants of the said Street should be assembled once a year in order to maintain a friendly intercourse amongst them, and particularly to inquire if any differences subsisted between any of them, and if there did any such difference exist, to use their friendly Offices to reconcile and Compose them. Accordingly this friendly meeting on Midsummer Eve in every year has subsisted beyond the memory of any man to this day June 23rd 1778.

"Mr. John Brecknell an unmarried man living in the Church Street in Kidderminster who dyed on the 7th day of March 1778 did by his last Will dated the 4th day of December 1776 bequeath the sum of One Hundred and Fifty Pounds to John Watson Nicholas Penn and William Lea in trust for the Inhabitants of the said Street to dispose of the Interest arising there from; in the following Words

Viz^t

Whereas there is a friendly Society or yearly meeting of Neighbours Inhabiting in the Church Street in Kidderminster on Midsummer Eve; Now for the better establishment and continuance of the said Friendly Meeting for Ever I do hereby give and bequeath to my faithful Friends John Watson Nicholas Penn and William Lea out of my personal Estate the sum of one Hundred and Fifty Pounds to be paid to them in One Month after my decease in Trust, to be by them placed out at Interest upon some Landed Estate or other good Security such as they or the major part of them shall approve and the Interest arising therefrom to be applied in manner following Viz^t to provide, and pay for, and give to every Child or unmarried Person that is born in or an Inhabitant of the Church Street aforesaid, One twopenny plumb Cake upon the Eve of every Midsummer Day - and further to provide and pay for Pipes Tobacco and Ale &c for the Entertainment of the Male Inhabitants which shall then Assemble - And the remaining part of the Interest arising from the above One Hundred and Fifty Pounds to be given to such poor Persons as the Company then Assembled or the majority of them shall think the fittest Objects; but it is my Will that no more than five shillings nor less than two shillings shall be given to any One And it is further my Will - that preference be always given to such poor Persons as are inhabitants in the said Street but never to be given to any one Person who is present at that Meeting And in order to perpetuate this Trust for Ever, it is my Will and I do hereby direct that whenever either of the Trustees before mentioned shall happen to dye or remove their Habitation out of the Church Street then the Inhabitants of the said Street who shall be assembled on Midsummer Eve next after such Death or removal shall Elect and choose some other Person Inhabiting in the Church Street to be a Trustee in the room and place of him who shall so dye or remove And so to Elect and choose in the room of any of the Trustees by me Appointed or of any Trustee hereafter Chosen as directed above as often as any such Trustee shall Dye or Remove and on for Ever. And it is my Will that if any of my Trustees now appointed or hereafter Chosen shall become Insolvent, or shall refuse to act or to account to the Inhabitants as aforesaid for the receipts of the Interest or shall so misbehave in their Trust as to offend the Inhabitants The said Inhabitants or the major part of them, Assembled as aforesaid shall have power under their Hands to discharge all or any of the said Trustees and to Elect choose and appoint other Trustee or Trustees to act in their place and stead. And it is my will that my Trustees shall not be answerable for any loss sustained by any insufficient Security or Securities so as the said loss be not sustained through their own wilful fault or neglect nor shall any of them be answerable for the fault or neglect of others of them.

"All the rest and Residue of his real and personal Estate he gave to his brother William Brecknell and appointed him Executor who paid into the hands of the Trustees the sum of One Hundred and Fifty Pounds, bequeathed as Above.

133

"Upon the 7th day of December 1776 Mr. John Brecknell made and published a Codicil to his Will in his own hand writing and left the further sum of One Hundred Pounds in the following Words

Viz^t

My further Will and desire is that my Executor shall in one Month after my decease pay into the hands of the Persons in Trust that is John Watson Nicholas Penn and William Lea the further sum of One Hundred Pounds to be disposed of by them in the following manner. That is first to cause to be erected over my Grave a Tomb in a plain manner; that is a Strong Stone laid upon Bricks &c what money remains after the Tomb is Erected desire the Trust will put it out to Interest upon Land Security and what money the Interest shall produce desire may be disposed of upon Midsummer Eve in the manner as mentioned in the foregoing part of my Will - I also give to the three persons above mentioned in Trust: five Guineas for to see the Tomb Erected and to settle a future distribution of the Bread and Money amongst the poor.

"The executor was informed that the above Legacy came within the Statute of Mortmain on account of the direction to put the money 'out to Interest upon Land Security' He therefore took Counsel's Opinion who advised him that he was not compellable to pay any more of the Hundred Pounds than the expense of Erecting the Tomb and accordingly upon Application he did refuse to pay any more than was sufficient for that purpose to the Trustees –

"The Will was proved at Worcester."

I have always been interested in the Church Street Supper and the Brecknell Charity. The first time I ever attended the supper was in 1883 and I have rarely missed one since. In 1892 I was appointed Secretary and one of the Trustees, and I held these offices until I moved from Church Street in 1937. My three children were born in the street and are therefore entitled to receive the loaves and cakes as long as they live, wherever they may be.

A minute book is kept of the proceedings at every meeting and this book is signed by every person present. There was no supper to begin with, only ale, pipes, and tobacco being provided at the meeting. The following resolution appears in the minute book as having been passed in 1903:-

> "That all the male householders resident in Church Street shall meet together at a common supper and that the sum of thirty shillings shall be paid to the host. That the supper shall be a plain supper and only beer and whisky shall be provided on the occasion."

> It was also agreed "That no one who is likely to be a recipient of the charity shall be invited to the supper."

There is never any difficulty in finding volunteers to act as hosts and give the supper, which cannot be provided from the small sum granted from the funds. At the meeting each year one of the residents volunteers to act as host the next year, and it has very often been a medical man. In addition to the residents in the street, the host usually invites the Mayor, the Vicar of the parish, and other prominent men in the town, as well as some of his personal friends. In the year 1918, and again in 1931, collections were made at the meeting to provide money for the reparation and re-painting of John Brecknell's tomb.

In the year 1907, when I was the host, Mr. J.G. Brecknell of Evesham, a descendant of Mr. John Brecknell, was present and his health was drunk. The Kidderminster Times published a report upon this, as follows:-

> "Mr. Brecknell, who was cordially received, returned thanks to Dr. Lionel Stretton for honouring him with an invitation to be present at the Brecknell Charity Supper this year. He said he heartily appreciated the kindness shown him and those gatherings of the residents of the old street interested him greatly. They seemed to become more interesting every year, and it was most gratifying to him to see so many people gathered together that night in honour of a relative of his whose desire was to promote peace, friendship and good neighbourhood. He hoped that all who

took part in that celebration would realise the value of those good qualities and try to practise them in their daily life and work. He also thanked Dr. Stretton for the able and honourable manner in which he had handled the charity, which was so interesting to him, and trusted it might remain in his hands for many years."

The following extracts are taken from the Kidderminster Times report of the Church Street Peace and Good Neighbourhood Supper of Midsummer Eve, 1924. They show that the wishes of the founders of the feast are carefully observed:-

"Under the general presidency of Dr. H. Lawford Miles, and attended by practically all the residents of Church Street - a highly-valued residential quarter of the Carpet Borough of Kidderminster - another successful celebration of the 'Peace and Good Neighbourhood' Charity took place on Midsummer's Eve and gave pleasure and profit to all who were permitted to be present.

"At 8 o'clock the company partook of supper, with Dr. Miles as 'mine host.' A short business meeting followed, at which the affairs of the charity were dealt with and settled for the ensuing year.

"Dr. Lionel Stretton, J.P., as the secretary to the charity, read the balance sheet, which showed that the interest on £275 worth of Consols at 3 per cent. was £6. 17s. 4d, plus 2s. to be added as the interest lent to the former chairman; total, £6. 19s. 4d. The loaves and cakes which had been distributed this morning cost £1. 10s. (as last year); the long pipes, ale, tobacco, etc. cost £2. 5s. 4d., leaving a balance of £3. 4s. to be distributed among people - widows - who resided in Church Street, to whom preference had to be given, and to one born in the street. Eleven persons had received 5s. each, and two 4s. 6d. each, which absorbed all the money.

"The Chairman, at the request of the Secretary, signed the book in token that the affairs of the charity had been duly dispensed in a satisfactory way, and in harmony with the terms of the trust, and then called upon the company to attest the accuracy of the record

136

by attaching their signatures. This, too, was done, all present signing the historic old book, which dates back about 150 years.

"The Chairman then put the usual formal question to the company - whether any difference subsisted between them; if so, it was his duty to try and compose any such differences. They would allow them an opportunity to permit of their adjusting any differences which might exist.

"After a pause, Dr. Miles, having received no response, took it that there was no sort of ill feeling or bad will subsisting between any of those present. He would now propose the old toast 'Peace and Good Neighbourhood' which was suitably received.

"The Chairman, replying to the vote of thanks proposed in a speech by the Secretary said that it had been the greatest pleasure in the world to him to be present that evening and entertain the company in a small way. He hoped the 'Peace and Good Neighbourhood' meeting would be continued for years and years, though, had it not been for their indefatigable Secretary, Mr. Stretton, the probability was that this old-world celebration would have fallen through many years ago."

The following is the main part of my speech at the meeting in the year 1925, when I myself was the host:-

"I thank you sincerely for the very cordial manner in which you have proposed and passed the vote of thanks to me. It has given me great pleasure to act as your host this evening, and if you have enjoyed the gathering as much as I have it is a good augury for the future maintenance of these meetings. I trust we may all be spared to come together in 'friendly intercourse' on many such occasions, and that the generations that follow us will never allow this agreeable and beneficial custom to fall into desuetude. Each generation should hand down the tradition to the next, as it was received by us from our forefathers.

"We know that the honour of having instituted this annual gathering belongs to a woman. We do not know her name; in the record in our book she is called simply 'a maiden woman'. Nor do

137

we know the date of the institution of the custom; it is lost in the mists of antiquity. It was probably generations - it may have been centuries - before the Brecknell bequest. To quote from our first record: 'This friendly meeting on Midsummer Eve in every year has subsisted beyond the memory of any man to this day June 23rd 1778.'

"A further quotation from our book states: 'It seems to be the principal intention of the original donor, that the male inhabitants of the said street should be assembled once a year in order to maintain a friendly intercourse amongst them, and particularly to inquire if any differences subsisted between any of them, and if there did any such difference exist, to use their friendly offices to reconcile and compose them.

"In accordance with the desire of our foundress I have already asked you whether any differences subsist between you. This question, familiar as it is to us, will well repay detailed examination. Unfortunately our language - and probably the same is true of other languages - is not always as explicit as it might be. Many of our words can have several and diverse meanings; consequently in order to find out what a particular word is intended to convey it is often necessary to refer to the context. The words 'difference' and 'subsist' are striking examples.

"Surely the old lady would not object to our having differences of opinion. We have different views and tastes; it would be a very peculiar and inconvenient world if we all thought alike. Suppose we all wanted to follow the same occupation, or to buy the same joint of meat! I consider that differences of opinion are very beneficial, and I do not see why they should lead to quarrels. But if you look up the word 'difference' in a good dictionary you will find that it means not only a disagreement of opinion but also a quarrel, and there can be no doubt that is the meaning intended here.

"Now what does the word 'subsist' mean? In one sense (though rather an unusual one) I have subsisted you tonight by providing you with a dinner; in another, slightly different and more common, sense, you are subsisting on the dinner: but neither of these meanings will suit our quotation. The dictionary gives yet another - to continue to exist - and that is obviously the correct meaning here. So that a difference subsisting means a quarrel that continues to exist. This detailed study of the English language is often necessary if we are to find out the real meaning of what we hear or read.

"A quarrel continuing is the bad thing that our foundress wished to put a stop to. A difference of opinion may be a good thing, but continuing quarrels are bad things; they are bad for individuals, for communities, for organisations of all descriptions, and for nations. They often lead to bloodshed and on occasions to the arbitrament of war: millions of innocent lives may be sacrificed in the settlement of the quarrel, and the so-called settlement often merely postpones the renewal of hostilities.

"I feel sure we are all agreed that it is very desirable to avoid personal strife, and we are pleased to know that this street at least is free from it.

"The Brecknell part of our meeting is of more recent origin than the other, and I cannot too often insist on the fact that the Church Street Supper and the Brecknell Charity are two distinct things, though our annual meeting commemorates them both.

"As I have already stated, honour for the original idea - original in both senses - is due to the 'maiden woman'; but to John Brecknell we must give the credit of recognising the excellence of the idea and of contributing to its development and extension by the bequest he made and his instructions regarding it.

"John Brecknell's will is dated the 4th of December, 1776. He died at the age of 66 on the 7th March, 1778, and was buried in a vault in St. Mary's Churchyard. The inscription on the tombstone reads as follows:-

To the Memory of William Brecknell
sen. Died 22 April 1764 age 72.
Also of Mary his Wife died 22 June 1766 age 89.
Susannah their Dau^r died 13 March 1766 age 54
John Brecknell their Son died 7 March 1778 age 66
Who left 150 to the inhabitants of Church Street.

"As you know, the conditions of John Brecknell's bequest have been faithfully carried out.

"In conclusion, I think I shall be voicing your own feelings if I express my opinion that we owe a debt of gratitude to our ancient benefactress. I am convinced that this annual gathering has been a source of great pleasure and benefit to the inhabitants of our street, and it has not been without influence beyond our boundaries.

"I have often uttered the wish that the happy conditions and 'friendly intercourse' subsisting among us could be annually celebrated in all parts of the town, in other towns, and among all races throughout the world. Especially desirable is such a consummation now that conversations are so frequently taking place between the nations. The world is weary of strife and would welcome the substitution of a just and lasting peace for the clash of arms, the party quarrels, the violence of class conflict, and the hatred and atrocities engendered and perpetuated by international warfare.

"Let us each and all do our share in working towards the attainment of this high ideal, so beautifully expressed in the words of the Russian National Anthem – 'Give to us peace in our time, O Lord!'

CHAPTER XIX

FASHIONS

Papers read. Natural Hegelians. Dress for women. Crinolines. Variety. Amount of clothing. Bicycling dress. Hair. Ornaments. Cosmetics. Smoking by women. Dress of males. Fashions in general. Summer Time. St. John Long. Quack practice. Fashions in diagnosis. Medicines. Influenza. Appendicitis. Gall-bladder. Tonsils. Pyorrhoea. Antiseptics. Sterilisation of skin. Multiple crazes. Diet. Individuals. Drink. Bleeding. Linseed poultice. Exercise and rest. Individualism.

This chapter follows the lines of a paper I read at the summer meeting of the Kidderminster Medical Society in 1926; it was published later in the same year in The Medical Officer. I read much the same paper at an annual meeting of the Hospital Nurses' League in 1935. The subject is a controversial one and I chose it for the summer meeting of the Medical Society in the hope that it might be of so much interest to the women present at the meeting that they would join in discussing it afterwards.

A.B. Walkley wrote as follows:-

"Women are natural Hegelians. They recognise instinctively that the vital principle is not a state of being, but of becoming, and 'signify the same in the usual way' by choosing a new hat once a week. Just think what the world would be like if woman were not various and mutable! If she wore her old hats like a man! If she were re-painted and re-decorated only once in seven years like a leasehold flat! If her skirts remained through the ages of one and the same length! We should lose all motive for looking out of windows and have no future to look forward to! Human life would be petrified and curiosity extinct!"

Dress has always fascinated women and no matter what effect was produced they have ever been devoted slaves to the fashion in vogue. I remember the enormous crinolines that were worn in the days of my youth. They were very ugly and a great impediment, but no man would have dared to say so at the time. I suppose they possessed some advantages, but I am not in a position to define them. Later there was a sort of half crinoline, called a tournure, and finally a so-called bustle, which gradually diminished in size until it ended in a sausage-shaped pad about 2 or 3 inches in diameter, which was fixed over the sacrum. I am told that in this present year of grace (1939) there is a tendency to revive the crinoline, at all events in certain classes and on some occasions. I can only hope that the fashion may not become a general one, and in these days of sporting and other activities I cannot think that it will.

I sometimes think it would be an advantage if some of our women were Spartan enough to disobey the commands of fashion and continue to dress in the style they prefer and that suits them; but since the dawn of human existence it has been dangerous to oppose public opinion, and the effects are seen today. Perhaps, however, it would be a rather ludicrous world if our womenfolk were dressed at will in the various fashions that have characterised different periods. It would be something like a continuous fancy-dress ball. Homogeneity has its advantages, including the delight of donning new garments with each change of fashion and the pleasure of a husband in bringing home to his wife a new toque or a fur wrap.

It is not only the shape and the colour of clothes that have to be considered. The amount of the naked body exposed to view is of more than ordinary importance. We have travelled a long way from the veil. The high-necked bodice and the long skirt have for the time being disappeared; sleeves are shortened or discarded altogether, and on certain occasions the backs of bodices are almost non-existent. I cannot think that bodices can be made much scantier or skirt much shorter - they have already become 'shorts' - because if they are there will not be anything left to dress. Let us hope that the next fashion will demand an increase in the quantity of material used; this would benefit the manufacturers and tend to promote modesty. The dress of the girls who ride about on bicycles nowadays is most indecent. They might almost as well be naked. But even nakedness seems to be fashionable in some

142

quarters, though I cannot believe it will ever become general. Knowing as we do the deformities and abnormalities that occur we should dislike it all the more.

To me, fashion in clothes is more understandable than the desire to vary the anatomy. So far as stays and boots are concerned the alteration in anatomical construction is an unavoidable consequence; but to cut off hair, which has been one of the glories and attractions of women in bygone ages, appears to me to be a voluntary mutilation of a beautiful body that was designed by One who is a more capable judge and creator of beauty than those who presumptuously desire to alter His design.

The practice of making holes in the ears for the purpose of wearing ornaments is on the wane, but I am told that a custom is arising of piercing the arms by a kind of half bangle that clips on with spikes, and that similar ornaments are designed for the ankles. I presume that stockings will be discarded when these anklets come into vogue, indeed, during the summer months nowadays bare legs are by no means an uncommon sight, and how very far from beautiful many of them are! Perhaps the barbarous custom of boring the nose will be introduced here, and if it is I predict that most women will wear rings through their noses. The minor efforts by means of paint and powder are much in evidence. Plucked eyebrows, darkened eyes, painted lips, finger-nails and toe-nails have no charm for me. Why not have some pictures of hieroglyphics painted and tattooed on the exposed parts of the body? Perhaps that may yet become the fashion.

Smoking by women is not really new. When I was a boy I used to see old women smoking short clay pipes. They evidently enjoyed it and perhaps it did not do them much harm. But the smoking of numerous cigarettes by young girls is certainly most harmful. Some of them smoke 20, 30, 40, or even up to 100 cigarettes a day - a most pernicious habit!

The dress of the male sex is also influenced to some extent by fashion, though less so than that of women, and those of us who have the courage to persist in donning a top hat and a turn-down collar are regarded as cranks. It is not a very severe penalty for consistency, and when the top hat comes into fashion again, as I am told it will, we shall be saved a change.

143

Fashions are not confined to questions of personal adornment. They pervade almost every department of life and have far more effect than is generally realised, being followed almost universally. People are like a flock of sheep; the one that starts through a gap in the hedge sets the fashion, and there are none left behind. Most of our fashions are initiated by individuals, but we are not free from the influence of politicians, who enforce their fashion by Act of Parliament, as is evidenced by the Summer Time Act. This may have advantages. Some people like it; some people would like any change. But it causes births and deaths to be registered on incorrect dates, which might lead to expensive legal proceedings. This reminds me of a tombstone erected in a country churchyard not far from here. The inscription on it stated that the deceased died on the 31st September. I called the Vicar's attention to it and I believe it has been altered, but it is open to question whether the death took place on the 30th September or the 1st October.

In my own profession fashion plays a very conspicuous part. It matters not whether he is a surgeon, a physician, or a general practitioner, whether he is a qualified man or an ill-educated charlatan, if he is Mr. Fashion the flock will gather round him, and whatever mistakes he may make no-one will believe anything against him. This is exemplified in the person of St. John Long, a quack who flourished in Harley Street just over 100 years ago and is said to have made an income of £15,000 a year. It is easy to understand that ignorant people can be gulled, but when we see crowned heads, members of the aristocracy, leaders of religion and law, and astute business-men, fall victims to the lure of the quack it is almost impossible to account for their stupidity. I am sorry to say that even some of the qualified members of the profession are guilty of quack practice. From a financial point of view there is no doubt it is a success, but I do not envy such men the secret contemplation of their false practices.

The rule of fashion extends also to the genuine practitioners, both diagnosis and treatment being affected by it. Unfortunately these fashions are communicated to the general public, often through the medium of the daily press. They are discussed in drawing-rooms, at dinner-parties, and in the public bars. At one time every ill is attributed to arteriosclerosis. When the interest in this wanes, intestinal intoxication takes its place and the advocates of various forms of treatment have an

144

opportunity for a conflict. Some kind of aperient becomes the fashion; at one time it is cascara; at another, paraffin; and others have their turn. The inventor of a new aperient could soon make a fortune; but they are mostly old ones rehabilitated. I remember the cascara craze. An uncle of mine was a physician in the West End of London. When I told him of the new aperient he mounted the steps in his study and brought down a shabby volume more than fifty years old - Pereira's Materia Medica - in which the drug was fully described. It had gone out of fashion, like the broad-brimmed hat, but it came back. I have an idea that an excellent new aperient will be discovered and become the fashion in the future. Perhaps it will be castor oil or Epsom salts.

The influenza fashion has persisted longer than most of them. The public are so fond of it, and the general practitioner finds it such a useful refuge. His patients insist on having a name for their complaint, and here it is. An increase of temperature with no knowledge of its cause - call it influenza. If it turns out to be enteric, it is gastric influenza; if pneumonia, influenzal pneumonia; influenzal scarlet fever, or appendicitis, or anything else. I may be called a sceptic, but when I hear of a patient suffering from influenza I say to myself - an increased temperature and the doctor does not know the cause of it. I do not blame him. The public insist upon a name; influenza sounds very well, and if my definition were attached to it, it would be very accurate.

Appendicitis has had its day. I mean the period when it was so much the fashion that many people in their anxiety to be in the swim considered it necessary to undergo an operation for the removal of their appendix. There is no doubt that many healthy appendices were removed. Some enthusiasts went to the length of advising the routine removal of the appendix from a child soon after birth. I have often been asked my opinion and I always reply that the Almighty knows far better than I do how to construct a body. I have no hesitation in saying that a man with a normal appendix is a better man than if he had none; if it is diseased the sooner he is rid of it the better.

It was a fashion at one time to remove the gall-bladder. I was told some time ago that the surgeons in London have now abandoned the practice. I told my informant that I had never begun it, because I felt sure the gall-bladder was put there for some good purpose.

An elaborate operation for the enucleation of tonsils is now in fashion. I regard it as an undesirable mutilation. A guillotine properly used will remove all that it is desirable to remove of a hypertrophied tonsil. It is wise to leave a portion of the gland, for we do not know exactly what the function of the tonsil is. Perhaps in the future it will become apparent that the complete removal of both tonsils is detrimental to the general health.

Then we come to pyorrhoea. It is sad indeed to think of the numbers of sound teeth that have been sacrificed on the altar of this fashion, and when the deluded victims find that the artificial substitutes cannot be compared with the originals they cannot get their old friends restored. With all due respect to the dentists, I am opposed to the wholesale extraction of teeth; I never part with a tooth until I am driven to do so.

In surgery various antiseptics come and go. I think it was during the war that a wonderful new antiseptic was discovered and named Eusol. My grandfather used it under the name of Liq. sodii chlor., and my father used it too in his early days, but it went out of fashion. Carbolic had a long innings and poisoned a considerable number of people. It was used in the spray that was introduced by Lister and had not a long fashion. Some surgeons find that carbolic damages their skin, so they use Biniod. of mercury, and this is detrimental to the skin of others. I am told that cyllin is the most efficacious bactericide at present known, and that is the only consideration that should count.

The fashion of sterilisation of the skin with Tincture of iodine B.P.[4] was set by me, and I suppose I might take pride in the fact that it has held the field for thirty years. It is certainly very efficient and I see no reason for displacing it. But many do not use it to the best advantage because they do not understand that previous washing of the skin prevents its full action.

When several fashions are added together it is enough to daunt the bravest, to say nothing of the effect on his pocket. Here is an example. A man went to consult a well-known and very fashionable physician. He

---

[4] See Addendum 1

had been sleeping badly; he had vague pains about his body and had lost weight. No definite physical signs were present. After examination the physician gave him a packet of cards: No. 1 directed him to consult an X-ray specialist and have his teeth radiographed; No. 2 directed him to consult a dentist and have the condemned teeth extracted. A sound tooth was removed; No. 3 directed him to consult an ear and throat specialist and have all the sinuses examined; No. 4 directed him to have an X-ray examination of the abdomen after a bismuth meal; No. 5 directed him to send specimens of his blood and his excretions for analysis and bacteriological examination; No. 6 directed that vaccines should be prepared if found desirable.

When the patient finally came to me he had followed all these various directions and had had some doses of vaccine, without any benefit. He was not any better - a fact that was of some importance to him, though it did not affect the various investigators. The poor chap was obviously worried, and a quiet talk with him disclosed the cause of his trouble and enabled me to give advice that soon produced an improvement in his condition. It was a case where the obvious had been overlooked in a search for the improbable.

Diet is not free from the influence of fashion. At one time it is the meat diet that is the craze; at the other extreme is the vegetarian. I have witnessed the ban on tomatoes, because they were supposed to cause cancer; on rhubarb, for fear it should produce vesical calculus. I could cite many other articles of diet that have been banned for a period. Not one of these fashions is based on scientific facts. They are mostly the opinions of individual members of the profession, and the more prominent a man is the more positive are his opinions, and the more eagerly are they taken up by the general public. Fortunately these fashions do not last long and those who have followed them are soon able to enjoy their varied diet again.

There is no doubt that each individual is a law unto himself in the matter of diet. I have known persons in whom roast chicken caused acute gastric trouble, whereas they could eat roast pork without feeling any ill effects. This diet question may be the origin of the saying, "Every man is a fool or a physician at forty years of age." Even at half that age most people should know what articles of diet disagree with them, and

147

these they should try to avoid. I use the word 'try' advisedly, because so many have a particular liking for the course that disagrees with them. They forget their past discomforts and cannot resist the temptation to enjoy the forbidden fruit.

The advice of a physician should not be based upon his knowledge of the effects of various articles of diet upon himself. He should learn the history of each patient and advise him accordingly, avoiding the narrow views and fads of cranks. But if there is a fashion in eatables, how much more is this evident in drinkables. At one time an excessive consumption of alcohol is advocated; at another, total abstinence. Tea, coffee, cocoa, even hot and cold water, all have their periods of fashion.

Among other treatments, bleeding had its day, when it was customary for healthy persons to have a pint or two of blood abstracted from their bodies at the barber's shop every spring and every autumn. That wholesale bleeding was a mistake few will deny, but the practice had its uses. It is still advantageous in some cases. I am told that abstraction of blood by the application of leeches is in vogue again. In my opinion bleeding can be more safely accomplished by means of a clean knife.

Even the domestic linseed poultice was discarded for a time, but I learn that it is returning to favour again. It was described as a nasty septic mess; if properly made it should be neither septic nor a mess, and I know from personal experience that it is far more effective than fomentations.

We get crazes for exercise and for rest, probably neither of them well advised. In an earlier chapter I referred to the views of an eminent London physician who, when asked his opinion of the prevailing craze for exercise, said he would not walk even from the front door to his Brougham if he could get someone to carry him. He was a small stout man, whom one might have imagined as a candidate for apoplexy, yet he lived to be eighty-three years of age.

In my profession we should never be swayed by fashion but always keep before us the fact that we are dealing with different individuals. What may be good for one is unsuitable for another, and it behoves us to keep in mind every fashion that has existed and to apply the one we consider the most likely to achieve the desired result.

CHAPTER XX

SOME EVENTS THAT MARK THE PROGRESS OF OUR LIVES

Introductory. Determination of sex. Ante-natal brain. Birth. Natural age limit. Happiness and misery. Ante-natal defects. Notification of birth. Registration. Names. Vaccination. Teeth. Circumcision. Tonsils and adenoids. A novel treatment. Early recollections. Christening and confirmation. Religion. Women's hair. Coming of age. Choice of work. Marriage. Marriageable age. Statutory minimum age. Early marriage. Limitation of families. Financial question. Education. Other events. Death. Right to die. Sudden death. Burial. Anthrax. Cremation. Post mortems. Towers of Silence. Controversial views.

It has sometimes been difficult to choose a subject suitable for a paper to be read at the summer meeting of the Kidderminster Medical Society, but this chapter is founded upon one I read in 1928. I purposely introduced some controversial matter in order to give my hearers an opportunity of stating and defending their own views if they were in opposition to mine.

There are certain definite events that mark the progress of our lives. Most of these events are common to all of us, though there is variation in their character and in the period when they occur; others are confined to the separate sexes. The first event is our conception, and with this is associated the determination of our sex. A great deal has been written about the determination of sex and some have ventured to state that it is under our control. Various methods have been suggested to determine sex - some of them have been tried - but there is no proof of their efficacy.

Most of us give our first kick about 4½ months after our conception. The time is not a fixed one, for some children are precocious and others are lethargic. This first kick raises the interesting question as to the earliest time at which a brain can function. It is produced by voluntary muscles, so that it should be under the control of the brain. The function of a pre-natal brain must be very limited and I cannot believe that the brain at this stage is capable of retaining any impression, though I believe it may receive one; it is certain that palpation of the mother's abdomen may, and sometimes does, cause a child to kick.

Our birth is an event of prime importance. To some children it may mean death; to others it may mean injury, in some instances so severe as to lead to permanent disability. Fortunately the majority of us have a safe passage into this world.

A normal child after birth may live for sixty or seventy years; some live for a longer period but very few will complete the century. There is probably a natural limit to human life; that limit has not been decided but I think it is somewhere between eighty and one hundred years. I have read in a book of some importance, "Man that is born of a woman hath but a short time to live and is full of misery." I am sorry I cannot agree with this statement. It would be equally true to say, "Man that is born of a woman hath a long time to live and is full of happiness." As I have often pointed out, relative terms convey no meaning to a scientific mind. I have no idea what "a long time" or "a short time" means, and probably a dozen people would give a dozen different interpretations of both these terms. And why should a man be full of misery or full of happiness? I do not believe that he can be full of either. The contrast is necessary. You cannot have happiness without a share of misery, nor can you have misery without a share of happiness. I admit that some individuals get a larger share than others - of both happiness and misery - and I have met some who make their misery a happiness. They appear to delight in grumbling about their ills and misfortunes, or, as is sometimes said, they are never happy unless they are miserable.

There are instances of ante-natal disease and of ante-natal accident. There are cases of faulty development. Some of the minor defects can be rectified by the surgeon, but others are so extensive that it is undesirable to keep the child alive. Our laws do not allow the right to kill and every effort is made to keep these undesirable children alive at the expense of their own suffering and the misery of their relations. Faults in

152

development are sometime attributed to maternal impressions. This view may be correct but the evidence is not convincing.

Within thirty-six hours of our birth we must be notified to the County Medical Officer of Health, a duty which is divided between the parents, the doctor and the nurse. This is a most unsatisfactory arrangement and it is surprising that notifications are not more often forgotten than they are. Within six weeks our birth has to be registered, and this is the duty of the parents. Before we are registered a name has to be chosen. It is a pity that we are not able to have any voice in the selection, because the names chosen by some parents cause the individual considerable inconvenience in after life. It is true that John Smith is not very distinctive, but John Lionel Stretton Smith is rather a mouthful; that is the name one of my Caesarean babies had to suffer from. But this sinks into insignificance by the side of Albert Grant Sir William Augustus Fraser Bart Smith, a name that was given to the son of parents who were enthusiastic politicians about fifty years ago. A businessman once told me that he had to sign his name eight hundred times in one day. Think what a labour it would have been for Albert Grant Sir William Augustus Fraser Bart!

If our parents are sensible we are vaccinated to protect us from small-pox. It is unfortunate that under our laws this precaution may be omitted. If the so-called conscientious objector himself paid the penalty of his folly I should not mind, but the dire consequences may fall upon his offspring at any period of his life, and the disease may spread with alarming rapidity and cause the loss of many lives.

We have to go through the process of cutting our teeth. Dentists can state the exact date at which each tooth appears, but the accuracy of their statements is sometimes nullified by infants who have their own ideas on the subject. I have known instances where they began the process ante-natally; I remember one baby that was born with five teeth. What a saving of anxiety it would be if all babies would follow this excellent example! Someone suggested that it would be a great blessing if we could be born with a set of artificial teeth; but he did not indicate what material they should be made of, and it would have to be a material that would be able to expand with the growth of the mouth.

Some babies are born with conditions that require operation. One mother asked me to "circumscribe" her son. Her request is worthy of Mrs. Malaprop, but her meaning is obvious. Most male babies are benefited by such an operation.

There is the question of enlarged tonsils and adenoids, which develop after birth. Many children are benefited by an operation; it may save them from ear, nasal, and other complications, provided that it is performed early enough. It is seldom that any individual reaches adult age without having enlarged tonsils removed, but I have removed them from patients aged 40 and 45 years. The tonsils can be effectually removed by an expert with the guillotine. I have already recorded my views on this matter.

The shortening event in a baby's life is of more importance to the mothers than to the surgeon. Dress is certainly of interest to them very early in life. I was attending a child about three years old; she was very ill and we could not get her to take notice of anything till her mother put on her cot a new pink frock. The child immediately sat up in her cot and asked to have the frock put on; then she began to take an interest in things and get better. This is a novel form of treatment that is worthy of consideration.

Of the early events, one of great interest is the first functioning of the brain. I have already suggested that it may act before birth. How far can we look back? This varies in different individuals. It has been stated that "Probably personal memory begins about four years old." This may be true of some persons, but others can remember farther back. Sir Walter Scott and Dr. Johnson are stated to have remembered events that occurred in their second year, and I have read that Macaulay had a curious recollection of the house his parents lived in when he was two and a half years old. It is difficult to prove these early recollections and it has been suggested that the person may have been told of the events in later life. It may be so sometimes, but some of the events are not important enough to be told in later life and yet they may have made an impression on the child's brain. I am positive I can remember riding in panniers: I can see the pony now in our garden, yet he was disposed of when I was eighteen months old.

Some of us are christened, and this ceremony is followed in due course by confirmation. A girl who was being interviewed by a prospective mistress was asked if she had been confirmed. "No," she replied, "I've had my appendix out and that's quite enough of operations for me." I am not well enough acquainted with all the religious bodies to know whether these ceremonies of christening and confirmation are common to all of them, but I feel most strongly that religion is one of the most important moral forces. I deeply deplore the differences that exist among religious bodies and the acrimonious disputes that sometimes take place between members of the same denomination. I believe these dissensions help to decrease the number of religious persons and weaken the influence that religion should exert.

Girls used to put their hair up at about 17 or 18 years of age. Most of them cannot do this now. I have already expressed my opinion about cutting the hair short. That I am not alone in my views is indicated by the result of the international beauty competition of the year 1928. The first prize was won by "Miss Chicago," the second by "Miss France," and the third by "Miss Italy," and all these three had long hair. I saw pictures of them in the Sketch.

We come of age - a time when some of us imagine that we suddenly achieve wisdom. It is true that coming of age confers upon us certain legal rights, but many persons are less capable at the age of 21 years than others are at the age of 16 years. Hard and fast rules with regard to age possess some advantages, but they lead to many hardships and errors. They try to eliminate individualism, which is impossible. Some persons are precocious. In the year 1928 a picture painted by a girl of fourteen was hung on the line at the Academy. This was all the more remarkable because she was said not to have received any lessons in painting. Truly an infant prodigy and if a prodigy in painting, why not prodigies in other respects?

Most of us have to choose our work in life. To some of us this choice presents no difficulty. I have known instances where children chose their future work at a very early age and never wavered from their decision. These are likely to be the most successful men. Some are incapable of arriving at a decision and this is one of the most difficult problems their parents have to face, because they may put the child into a position that will never be congenial to him.

Some of us get married. It was a speech I was asked to make at a wedding reception that suggested to me the idea of the paper on which this chapter is based. I feel very strongly that marriage is the most important event in our lives, and it should be the happiest. To say that the relations between man and wife are different nowadays is nonsense. The happiness of married life depends today, as it always has depended and always will depend, upon mutual love and affection. Some women have found fault with the promise to obey in the marriage service. I am told that the word 'obey' is now omitted, and for that very reason many girls are insisting upon saying it. How like them! If a girl loves the man she is going to marry - and no girl should marry a man unless she does love him - she will wish to obey him; and if a man loves the girl he marries he will never ask her to do anything she objects to doing.

It is true that there are a certain number of unhappy marriages, and it is also true that the number of divorces has increased since the obtaining of them has been made easier, but I believe that the great majority of marriages are happy. Of course you cannot have it all one way; there must be contrast. A man once told me how happy he had been with his wife. "We have been married over forty years," he said, "and we have never had a cross word." My reply was, "Poor fellow! What a lot you have missed! If you have never had a cross word you do not know what marital happiness means." My mother was the most affectionate wife and mother, and she and my father were lovers to the end. She was full of wisdom and gave me the best advice. Before my marriage she said to me, "Of course you will have quarrels with your wife. It is natural that you should. But never go to sleep until you have made them up." That was wise advice.

There is a great diversity of opinion about the age at which matrimony should be undertaken. It is unwise to decide upon a definite age, because persons differ so much. Some girls of 18 are more fit to be married than others are at 25, and some men of 25 are quite unfit to undertake the responsibilities of matrimony. Every marriage must be judged by the man and woman concerned, but I feel confident that early marriage is good for health and increases the happiness of life. I do not

156

go to the length of advising marriage at the age or 12 or 14, and I was astonished to find that the statutory minimum age of marriage in Great Britain is 12 years for girls and 14 years for boys. In 1927 a deputation waited upon the Home Secretary to try to get this statutory minimum age raised to 16 years for both sexes. I agreed with this, but my opinion was altered when the Home Secretary pointed out that the difficulty was that in the majority of cases of girls under 16 years who married there were urgent reasons for the marriage, and in the present state of public opinion there would perhaps be an outcry against disallowing marriage to young persons in such circumstances.

I think many girls of 18 or 19 years and many men of 22 or 25 years may be well fitted for matrimony, which includes the ability to decide upon their mates. To say that a girl should not be married early because she has not yet had what is called "a good time" is absurd. I aver that she can have a good time and a happy time in her own home, bringing up a family. To call this drudgery is altogether wrong. It should be the greatest possible joy, and that joy should be shared by the husband, whose duty it is to help his wife in every way that he can. Motherhood is more easily accomplished after an early marriage and young people find it easier to adapt themselves to each other than do those of maturer years.

The question of the limitation of families is too large a subject to be fully dealt with here. But I should like to point out that it is a question of international importance rather than of individual convenience. If England is to limit her population while other nations increase theirs how are we to hold our Empire together? Our Colonies demand more people, and if we do not provide them other nations will, and we shall be powerless to prevent their introduction into our Colonies and the probable consequent development of international complications.

It is appalling to know how the number of children has decreased of late years. The only encouragement given by the Government to those who would increase the number of their children is a rebate of income tax, but this rebate is not enough to induce parents to bring up larger families.

It is appalling to me too to read about the activities of those women who busy themselves in urging people to curtail the size of their families and in doing all they can to spread a knowledge of birth control. In my opinion these busybodies would be better occupied in bringing up families themselves. It has been stated that the time is approaching when the world will be over-populated. That may be so in the distant future but I do not believe that the time for necessary limitation of the population, has yet arrived.

The financial question looms large in the consideration of matrimony, as it did when I was young. "Our income is not large enough to enable us to live comfortably," say the young people. By comfortably they usually mean living in the style they have been brought up to; that is, they want to begin where their parents left off. I maintain that it is an excellent lesson in life to begin at the bottom rung of the ladder and work upwards. I do not advocate marriage on means insufficient for existence, but there is no need for motor-cars and champagne. Nor need those about to marry worry about the education of a family, which is another reason often advanced against early marriage. "We could not do well enough for our children," they say. It is not the duty of parents to provide for their children after they are grown up. Most men are happier if they have to earn their own living. I very much doubt whether it is a good investment to spend money on expensive schools. Education is not comprehended in what we learn at school, and provided that a child has a good grounding and has learnt the habit of work there is nothing to prevent his future success.

Other events that may enter into our lives include our successes and failures in our avocations, the attainment of wealth or social position, the part that we may play in public life and politics, the honours that may be bestowed upon us, the benefits that we may confer upon humanity by scientific discoveries, by inventive genius, by literary, artistic, or other gifts. But these are not common to all of us and it would be beyond the scope of this chapter to examine them in detail. I will therefore pass on to the final event:-

"Thou know'st 'tis common; all that lives must die. Passing through nature to eternity."

It is probable that few people reach the natural limit of human life. Many die in early life, but it is satisfactory to know that the average duration of life in this country has increased. This does not mean that the natural limit of life has increased. The improved average is due largely, if not entirely, to the lessened infant mortality.

The actual passing away is not necessarily a painful process; it may even be pleasant. William Hunter when on his deathbed is reported to have said, "O for the strength that I might write down how pleasant a thing it is to die!" I have been told of a man who said when he was dying that he had no idea it would be so pleasant.

Some diseases cause so much suffering that death is a welcome relief, and I cannot too strongly insist that those who suffer in this way should be given everything that can mitigate their pain. I cannot understand the mental outlook of those who express the opinion that it is wrong to give morphia to a patient suffering from a painful and incurable disease. Not only ought morphia to be given but it ought to be repeated and the dose increased to an amount that will keep the patient comfortable. It has to be a very large dose sometimes.

Whether human beings should have the right to terminate their own sufferings or whether others should have the right to kill are very serious questions. Much attention was drawn to a case where a father, overwrought with watching the sufferings of his child, placed her in a bath and caused her death. He was tried for murder and acquitted. The judge in his charge to the jury said that if the child had been one of the lower animals and the father had kept it alive to suffer he could have been punished. I put a similar argument forward in a paper I read many years ago, but I feel very strongly that a decision of such magnitude should not be left to any individual. I have often said that there are things that are worse than death, and one of them is life in a lunatic asylum. Anyone can be shut up in an asylum on the certificate of two doctors, so why should not a certificate from two doctors be considered enough to justify the termination of the life of a sufferer?

Though the actual process of death may be happy, the parting from dear relations and friends cannot fail to cause distress to all. In our Church Service we pray to be delivered from sudden death. It is the happiest ending we can have, but it often causes more distress to those who are left behind because it is a great shock to them. I always try to comfort them by pointing out that their dear one has been spared the pain of parting from them. Some clergy tell us that sudden death means unprepared death. Even so, I should not fear it, because I feel confident that we shall be judged by the lives we have lived and that a deathbed repentance will have little, if any effect upon our future condition.

After death comes the question of the disposal of the body. The elements of which it is composed must return to the crust of the earth from which they were derived. So far as I am aware there are three methods of disposal of the dead: (1) burial, (2) cremation, (3) the Tower of Silence. Burial is the method most in favour in this country. When the body is put in a coffin and buried in the earth the process of dissolution is said to occupy about fourteen years; if lead coffins and vaults are used dissolution may be delayed for a much longer period. What possible advantage can there be in delaying the return of our elements to the crust of the earth for such a long period when it can be accomplished in a couple of hours by means of cremation?

It is questionable whether burial may not cause harm to the living. We know that in some cases it has caused disease. An animal died of anthrax and was buried. Twenty years later an outbreak of anthrax occurred on the farm where this animal was buried and the disease was traced to the animal by the discovery of anthrax germs in the worm-heaps on the surface of the ground under which it had been buried. Now the Board of Agriculture insist upon the cremation of all animals that have died of anthrax. Yet the burial of human beings who die of anthrax is still allowed. If there is danger from the bodies of lower animals, surely there is danger also from the body of a human being.

Some people object to cremation for various reasons, one being that they imagine it is an expensive method of disposal of the dead. This is incorrect; cremation costs less than a burial. When the cremation is over about 97% of the body has gone up the chimney, so why deprive the crust of the earth of the remaining 3%? It is better to scatter the remaining ashes on the ground than to keep them in an urn. At most crematoria there is a so-called Garden of Rest where the ashes are scattered and where mourners can sit and contemplate.

160

Some think cremation might encourage crime, but I believe it would have the opposite effect. Before a cremation the death must be certified by the doctor in attendance; the body must be examined by an independent doctor, who must also give a certificate, and these two certificates must be submitted to a third doctor. There is no risk of being cremated alive.

In my opinion every dead body should be subjected to a post-mortem examination; the Registrar-General's statistics would then be of more value. These examinations should he made after the committal in a room adjacent to the incinerating chamber. The relatives should have the privilege of nominating a doctor to witness the examination and the incineration.

The Eastern custom of placing bodies on the Tower of Silence to be devoured by vultures is too repulsive for consideration, yet I can imagine that its advocates would prefer it to the process of decay that goes on in a grave.

Throughout this chapter I have used the various events of our lives as a series of texts about which I have stated my own views. These views are the outcome of long experience and serious thought, but I am quite aware that some of them would meet with considerable opposition both from members of my own profession and from the general public.

CHAPTER XXI

THE KIDDERMINSTER AND DISTRICT GENERAL HOSPITAL

Years on Staff. Comparison of Staff, 1882 and 1939. Dispensary. Infirmary. New building, 1871. Training of Nurses. War years. Army Council certificate. Extensions, 1926. Nursing Home and field adjoining. Statistics.

It may be considered that all voluntary hospitals are very much alike, though they may have some points of difference. This is so far true as to make it superfluous to give any detailed description of The Kidderminster and District General Hospital. This hospital has, however, played so large a part in my life and my professional career that it may not be out of place to give a short account of it. One general point may be mentioned at the outset: this hospital has a reputation for surgery, the amount and the variety of its surgical work being greater than are usually to be found in general hospitals of a similar size.

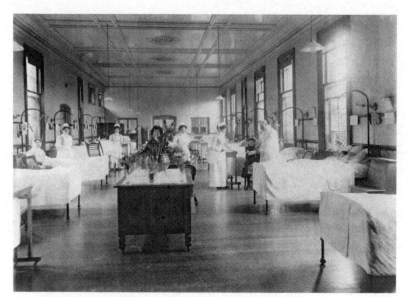

Kidderminster & District General Hospital – general surgical ward
Courtesy of Kidderminster NHS Treatment Centre

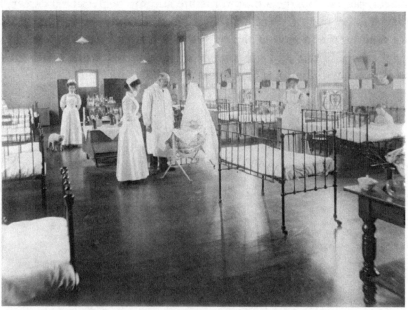

Kidderminster & District General Hospital – children's ward
Courtesy of Kidderminster NHS Treatment Centre

I succeeded my father as an honorary surgeon in the year 1882 and remained an active member of the Staff until my resignation at the end of 1938. I now hold the position of honorary consulting surgeon. When I joined the Staff there were four honorary surgeons, one house-surgeon, and five nurses. At the present time (1939) the honorary medical staff has nineteen members, there are two house-surgeons, and the nursing staff numbers fifty-four. The hospital has eight special departments.

A man could hardly spend fifty-six years in the continuous service of the same institution - be it hospital, bank, or what you will - without acquiring an intimate knowledge of that institution and a feeling that it is a part of himself. Throughout those fifty-six years I watched the growth and development of the hospital, and in the fourteen years, from 1924 to 1937, when I was its President I was also immediately concerned with the administrative side while at the same time carrying on my surgical work.

The history of this hospital, like that of most others, has been one of gradual growth, the development having been particularly marked during the last twenty-five years. The origin of the institution can be traced back to a Dispensary instituted in 1821. The next step was the establishment about the year 1850 of an Infirmary where in-patients could be received. In 1868, largely owing to the efforts of my father, who had been on the staff since 1857, it was decided to build a hospital worthy of the town, on a healthy site and planned in accordance with modern requirements. This new building was opened in 1871. At later periods an operating theatre, a mortuary chapel, an X-ray department, and many other improvements were added. About 1895 the hospital began a system of training nurses and in 1922 it was approved by the General Nursing Council for England and Wales as a First Class Training School for Nurses.

The high-lights in the history of the hospital may be said to be the period of the war and the opening of the extensions by His Royal Highness the Duke of York in 1926.

During the war the thirty beds placed at the disposal of the 1st Southern General Hospital for seriously wounded soldiers were kept continuously full, most of the patients receiving active surgical treatment.

Over 500 soldiers were treated, in addition to the civilian patients. The large amount of extra work involved was willingly undertaken and efficiently performed by the depleted staff. During this period a number of ladies, wishing to become efficient nurses, worked at the hospital as Special Probationers, paying for maintenance and giving their services. They were instructed by the Matron and afterwards proved themselves a credit to their training and of value to the nation.

In 1920 the Army Council sent the hospital the following certificate, signed by Winston S. Churchill. This has been framed and now hangs in the hall:-

> "During the Great War of 1914 - 1919 this building was established and maintained as a Hospital for British sick and wounded: the Army Council in the name of the Nation thank those who have rendered to it this valuable and patriotic assistance in the hour of its emergency, and they desire also to express their deep appreciation of the whole-hearted attention which the Staff of this Hospital gave to the patients who were under their care: the War has once again called upon the devotion and self-sacrifice of British men and women, and the Nation will remember with pride and gratitude their willing and inestimable service.

> "This certificate is presented by the Army Council, as a permanent record of their thanks, to be placed in the building which has been known and used as the Kidderminster Infirmary Hospital for British sick and wounded during the Great War, 1914 - 1919."

In 1924, the first year of my presidency, I launched an appeal for £25,000 to provide urgently needed extensions to the hospital, which serves a population of about 40,000, including Kidderminster and the surrounding districts. In two years, as the result of this appeal, we had received nearly £27,000 and in addition, more than £5,000 for endowment and upkeep. The commemoration stone of the new building was laid on August 13th, 1925, by Mrs. Stanley Baldwin (now the Countess Baldwin of Bewdley) as Deputy for her husband, the Right Honourable Stanley Baldwin, M.P., Prime Minister (now the Earl

Baldwin of Bewdley), who was summoned to London that day on urgent affairs of State.[5]

On July 21st, 1926, the extensions were opened, free of debt, by His Royal Highness the Duke of York, whose visit called forth an enthusiastic display of loyalty from the large crowds assembled to welcome him and to watch the ceremony.

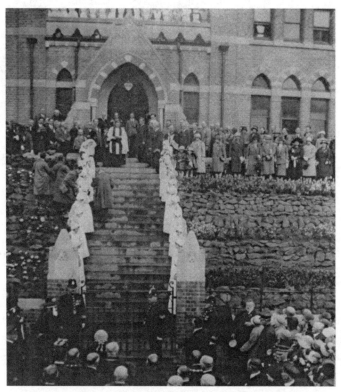

Kidderminster & District General Hospital extensions
Official opening by H.R.H. The Duke of York, K.G.
21st July 1926
Courtesy of Kidderminster NHS Treatment Centre

---

[5] See Addendum 4.1

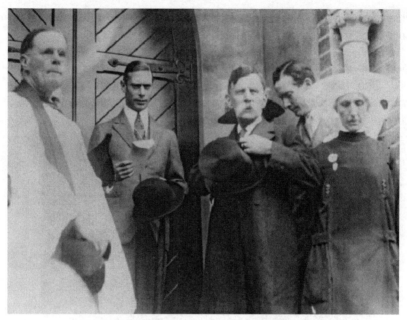

H.R.H. The Duke of York, K.G. – with envelope
John Lionel Stretton – with top-hat
Courtesy of Kidderminster NHS Treatment Centre

In a letter dated July 22nd, addressed to the President, His Royal Highness's Equerry wrote:-

> "The Duke of York was very much impressed by the new wing which has been added to the Kidderminster Hospital. His Royal Highness well realises the amount of work required to carry out this undertaking and it gave him the greatest pleasure to declare the building open."

The extensions included two new children's wards, containing forty cots, a new women's ward, with twelve beds, a new out-patient department and a laundry equipped with modern machinery. His Royal Highness the Duke of York gave us permission to name one of the children's wards the Princess Elizabeth Ward. The other we named the Stanley Baldwin Ward, because in 1918 Mr. Baldwin had provided the nucleus of the extensions scheme by a gift of £5,000. This gift was a thank-offering for twenty-five years of happy married life, and its object was the provision of a new children's ward as soon as the work could be undertaken, Mr. Baldwin's daughter having worked in the old children's ward during the war years.

The work of the hospital does not stand still, and so much has it increased since the year 1926 that a further extension of fifty more beds is now required. I had intended bequeathing my private Nursing Home to the hospital, but so strongly was I impressed with the urgent necessity for further development that in 1936 I presented the Home with its equipment to the hospital, on the sole condition that it should be kept up as a Nursing Home for paying patients. At the same time I gave a field adjoining the Hospital and the Home, with the intention that it should provide the site for the erection of the new wards required.

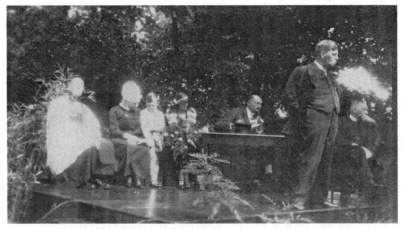

Lionel opening new wing of the nurses' home – 1931

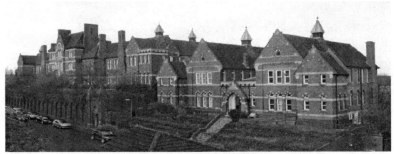

Kidderminster & District General Hospital and extension
2011 - Now converted to residential flats

The following striking statistics are enough to show how the work of the hospital has increased:

	1881	1921	1938
Number of beds	40	80	145
Number of in-patients	174	1,118	2,145
Average daily number of in-patients	15.6	54.69	114.57
Number of out-patients	1,496	696	5,521
Number of operations	18	1,067	3,210
Daily average of household	7.93	41.48	104.41

CHAPTER XXII

MY SEVENTIETH BIRTHDAY

A friendly ceremony. An unexpected tribute. Gratitude and appreciation.

Few events in my life have given me more pleasure and have touched me more deeply than a friendly little ceremony that took place at the hospital on the 20th September, 1930, the seventieth anniversary of my birthday.

I arrived at the hospital, as was my daily habit, at 10 o'clock in the morning, put my top hat in its usual place in the hall, and was about to begin my work of seeing out-patients and going all round the wards. To my astonishment the Matron asked me to go to the Board Room, and there I found a gathering of as many of the resident staff as could be spared to attend. I was entirely unprepared for what was coming, for the secret had been well kept. On the table was a handsome silver cigar box, inscribed simply with the initials J.L.S. and the date, September 20th, 1930. The Matron read the following:-

"Dear Sir,

The House-Surgeon, the Nursing and Domestic Staffs, the Dispenser, the Masseuse, the Office Staff, and the Collectors, ask you to accept this cigar box as a small token of love, honour, and affection on this, the seventieth anniversary of your birthday.

You have always given freely and ungrudgingly of your time, your talent and your health (and of your wealth) for the benefit of your fellow-creatures. The example set to all has been a high one, and it has been the aim of each one of us to try to attain the standard thus set before us.

It may hearten you to know that all, including the kitchen staff and the porters, were anxious to give something towards the gift for our President and Senior Honorary Surgeon, in fact to 'Father' (which is a term of endearment and respect), who is the friend of us all.

I have pleasure, Sir, in asking you to accept this small gift with our best wishes for many, many happy returns of the day."

I was so overwhelmed that I found difficulty in expressing my feelings adequately. I assured my hearers that I was very grateful for all the kind words that had been said to me, that I very much appreciated the beautiful present given to me by my own Staff in the field of their and my own daily work, and that I should treasure the gift as one of my most valued possessions and hand it down to my family as an heirloom. I said that I could hardly believe that I was seventy, for I did not feel seventy. I was thankful that I could still take the same keen interest in my work and do it as well as ever.

I concluded by saying that I should have more to say to the Nursing Staff on a forthcoming occasion, when the Nurses' League would be inaugurated; in the meantime I asked all those present to accept my heartfelt thanks for this cheering evidence of their loyalty and affection.

My remarks were received with loud and prolonged applause and as I left the room and went along the corridor to begin my daily work I was followed by the sound of enthusiastic cheers, called for and led by the Assistant Matron.

CHAPTER XXIII

FIFTY YEARS ON THE HOSPITAL STAFF: 1882 – 1932

Fifty years. Nurses' League. Management Committee. Honorary Medical Staff. Meeting of Governors. Gratitude for tributes.

In December, 1932, one of the years of my Presidency, I completed fifty years of service on the Honorary Medical Staff of the Hospital[6]. This being a somewhat rare event, I received many gratifying tributes and presentations, which will be recorded in this chapter in the order of the date on which these tributes were paid. I shall not attempt to give a full account of my various speeches of thanks on these occasions.

The annual meeting of the Hospital Nurses' League was held at the Nurses' Home on the 30th November, 1932. I had been specially invited to the meeting and found a very warm welcome awaiting me. The Matron said:-

> "As you all know, the special purpose of our meeting this afternoon is to show our respect and affection for our President, who in December, two or three weeks hence, will have been fifty years on the Staff of the Hospital. We felt that we could not let this opportunity go by without giving him some proof of our respect and affectionate regard. We ask him to accept this gift from past and present members of the Nursing Staff, the Masseuse, the Dispenser, the Secretarial Staff, and the present

---

[6] See Addendum 4.2

Domestic Staff. We wish him every happiness and that he may go on for another fifty years."

The gift was a very beautiful old Georgian silver coffee-pot.

The monthly meeting of the Management Committee held on the 14th December, 1932, corresponded to the meeting at which I had been appointed on the Staff fifty years before. As President of the Hospital, I was in the Chair. At the beginning of the meeting the Chairman of the House and Finance Committee rose and spoke as follows:-

"Before we start on the ordinary business of this meeting there is one matter that I should like to refer to, and I think it is only fitting that we should refer to it. I understand that in December, 1882 - fifty years ago - the Management Committee passed a resolution appointing Mr. J. Lionel Stretton a member of the Honorary Staff.

"I think I may say that when Committees pass such resolutions they do it hoping for the best. But I feel sure that no-one on that Committee could have imagined that that resolution would have such a remarkable result as fifty years of service from the member they then appointed. I doubt whether such a record has ever been equalled in any hospital in this country, and I feel sure it has certainly never been surpassed. The number of people that Mr. Stretton has treated in those fifty years must be more than the total number of the population of the town today.

"But Mr. Stretton's service has been not only on the medical side. I think we ought to realise and to say that he has been the moving spirit in the administration of this Hospital. He has helped it to develop from small beginnings into the Hospital we have today, and he has brought it not only to the size but also to the state of high efficiency that modern hospitals must reach if they are to meet the needs of the population. The extensions and developments throughout these years have been very considerable and they have been carried out in a manner that is second to none in this country.

"I feel that we should express to Mr. Stretton our very deep thanks and our great appreciation of the service he has given to this Hospital not only on the medical side but also on the administrative side. We wish him many more years of health and happiness in the continuation of his work. I have very great pleasure in proposing this resolution of thanks and good wishes."

The Chairman of the Hospital Saturday Fund Committee then said:-

"I have much pleasure in seconding this resolution. If Mr. Stretton had completed fifty years of service on one of the firms in the town he would probably have been presented with a nice gold watch. But the people of Kidderminster would have been very much worse off if his activities had been in that direction. For Mr. Stretton has been the surgeon and the adviser of the suffering poor, and he has given them fifty years of gratuitous service. Mr. A. mentioned a number equal to the present population of Kidderminster, but I think if we added another 50 per cent we should be nearer the mark. For in addition to Mr. Stretton's 40,000 operations he has given advice and medical treatment to great numbers of patients. Imagine if you can what a huge amount of suffering he has cured or relieved. I do not quite know how to express these things. An architect or a builder can see and rejoice in the buildings he has created, and they can be seen by others. The good work done by a doctor is not to be seen in the same way. But the remembrance of it lives in grateful hearts. I know that Mr. Stretton's noble, self-sacrificing work for fifty years is remembered by many grateful hearts and I hope that this does repay him in some measure.

"Kidderminster ought to be proud of her citizen. Kidderminster will have to lose him one day, and not till then will the value of his life and work be fully realised. This Institution has grown from small beginnings into the important Hospital we have today, and most of this has been the work of our President.

"I have very great pleasure in seconding the resolution. We hope that Mr. Stretton will live for very many years more in

175

comfort and good health, and that for many years more he may be able to continue his valuable work."

Other members of the Committee then added tributes, as follows:-

Mr. B. "I have reason to be grateful to Mr. Stretton. Forty-five years ago he operated on my arm and but for his skill and care I should have lost it, and perhaps my life too."

Mr. S. "I also have great reason for gratitude for all that has been done for my wife. Some few months ago one of the Sisters here told me that the people of Kidderminster did not realise what they had got in Mr. Stretton and they would not realise it until they had lost him. She said she had worked in hospitals all over the country and she had never before met a surgeon like Mr. Stretton; he would come at any hour of the day or night and do the most difficult and delicate operations with such skill and apparent ease and without any fuss or bother. His quiet manner in itself was enough to inspire confidence in patients and nursing staff."

The Treasurer of the Hospital. "I wish to say that the same sentiments as have just been voiced are expressed in the letters I receive from the general public. Our very deep and grateful thanks are due to our President for his services during these fifty years."

The resolution was carried with acclamation.

On the 3rd January, 1933, the Honorary Medical Staff held a meeting at which they paid me the following tribute. The meeting was presided over by the Senior Physician, the Chairman of the Staff Committee, who said:-

"Gentlemen, as you know, Mr. Lionel Stretton has recently completed half a century as Surgeon to this Hospital, and we have met to show recognition of this fact. We understand that during that period of fifty years he has performed some 40,000 operations. We do not know how many valuable lives he has saved, nor how much suffering he has relieved, but surely the total must be a very large one. If we consider it from a lower basis, the financial one, a ridiculously small fee of one guinea per operation

176

makes £40,000 and more, and a moderate average fee of five guineas per operation means nearly a quarter of a million of money, so that we may say he has made a gift of that amount to the poorer inhabitants of our town and neighbourhood. What a generous gift!

"And he is still going strong. His hand has not lost its cunning nor his natural force abated.

"John Lionel Stretton, On behalf of your colleagues on the Hospital Staff I have the honour, and the very great pleasure, of asking your acceptance of this fruit dish and flask as an expression of their appreciation of the work you have done in and for this Hospital during the last fifty years, and as a token of the feelings of esteem and affection with which they regard you.

"May this dish be filled with 'rare and refreshing fruit' and may the contents of this flask serve to comfort and revive you in times of stress and weariness!

"This address has been prepared for me by Mrs.-- as follows:-

> 'Presented to John Lionel Stretton on completion of fifty years devoted service as Surgeon to the Kidderminster and District General Hospital by his colleagues on the Honorary Medical Staff. December, 1932.'

and I am asking all the subscribers, that is all the members of the Medical Staff, to sign it.

"Mr. Stretton is very familiar with the unpleasantness of collecting subscriptions, but I can assure him that in this instance there was no unpleasantness, but very much the reverse; all were ready, even eager, to subscribe.

"I should mention that there is one subscriber who is not a member of the Staff - the Director of the Wellcome Museum of Medical Science, who visited the Hospital some three years ago in connection with Mr. Stretton's pathological specimens. He writes:

'Enclosed is a small cheque which you can apply in any way you like to express my appreciation of a really great man.'"

The fruit dish was an exceptionally beautiful silver one.

At the Annual Meeting of the Governors of the Hospital on the 14th March, 1933, tributes were paid to my fifty years of work by the Mayor, the Deputy Mayor, the Chairman of the Medical Staff Committee of the Hospital, and others, and a presentation was made to me. The personal gift took the form of a handsome silver salver of Chippendale style, bearing the following inscription in Caslon type of the same period:-

> 'Presented to J. Lionel Stretton, Esq., J.P., by the friends and supporters of The Kidderminster and District General Hospital on the occasion of his completing fifty years as a member of the Honorary Medical Staff, in recognition of the long, devoted and valuable services rendered to the people of this Town and District. 1882 – 1932.'

On the same occasion the following letter, signed by the Honorary Treasurer of the Hospital, was handed to me:-

> "Dear Mr. Stretton, In response to the very generally expressed desire to recognise your valued services to The Kidderminster and District General Hospital throughout the last fifty years, the sum of £1752. 16s. 11d. has been credited to the account of the Hospital.

> "May I, at the same time, express my personal hope that you will, for many years to come, be enabled to continue those services which, both from the medical and administrative side, have done so much for the Institution and for the sick and suffering of the district. Yours faithfully, —Treasurer."

The cheque was the outcome of an appeal made by the Mayor to commemorate my fifty years' service by an attempt to wipe out the balance of the debt incurred in 1931 by the building of a new wing to the Nurses' Home and extensions to and re-equipment of the kitchen department of the Hospital.

The speeches I made on these four separate occasions followed much the same lines. The meetings with my colleagues on the Staff and with the Nurses' League were particularly moving occasions. When speaking to them I stressed the point that the highest tribute a man can receive is a tribute from those he has worked with and I expressed my profound appreciation of that tribute. In all the speeches I said I fully recognised that surgery was a team job and that I owed a deep debt of gratitude to all the members of the team who had helped me in my work: my colleagues on the Staff, House-Surgeons, Matrons, and our efficient Nursing Staff. I also said I felt that the tributes paid to me should be paid to my father and mother, for it was they who had inspired me with love for the Hospital and the desire to serve my fellow-men with all the powers at my command. I expressed the hope that I might be able to continue my work for a few years longer and said it would be my greatest pleasure to do all I could to relieve the sufferings of those who needed help.

I assured my hearers of my gratitude for all the kind words spoken about me and for the beautiful gifts I had received, which would be constantly used and treasured as valued possessions to be handed down in my family as heirlooms.

CHAPTER XXIV

HOUSE-SURGEONS

Keen House-Surgeons. Advantage of small hospital. Successes. Temporary insanity. Incident at hotel. Instant discharge. Suicide. Cocaine. Trying career.

I have had a great deal of experience with House-Surgeons. The Kidderminster and District General Hospital has been fortunate in having the services of some extremely capable young men, English, Scottish, and Irish, trained in some of the leading hospitals of the three countries. Some of the best of these House-Surgeons have applied for re-appointment when the period of their service came to an end, because they realised that this hospital gave them exceptional opportunities of extending their knowledge and gaining varied experience. It is well known that a House-Surgeon who is keenly interested in his work will probably get greater experience in a comparatively small hospital than in a very large one, especially if the smaller one does many kinds of work and a great deal of surgery. In the smaller hospital he will see something of, and take part in, most kinds of medical and surgical work; in the larger one he is more likely to be limited to certain departments of the work.

Some of the former House-Surgeons of this hospital have attained important positions and many of them have established flourishing private practices, both in this neighbourhood and elsewhere.

The first House-Surgeon I remember at the hospital was there when I was a child. He once went temporarily off his head and had to be taken to an asylum. One day I was sitting in my father's carriage at the door of the hospital and another carriage and pair was waiting to take the House-Surgeon away. He came out of the door, got into my father's carriage, took off his hat and began to sing to me. Nothing would move him out

181

of that carriage. My father had to come and sit by him and drive with him through the town, while all the time he continued his singing. The other carriage followed us until we got a few miles away from the town, when at last the House-Surgeon was persuaded to get out of our carriage and into the other. He recovered completely and did quite well in later life.

Among the numbers of House-Surgeons I have known, many of them excellent, it is not surprising that a few have been unsatisfactory in one way or another. Two or three of them ended by committing suicide.

One very capable House-Surgeon, who had been trained at one of the leading hospitals, afterwards went to practise in South Wales, and some years later I saw in a newspaper the announcement of his death. He had gone from home to stay the night in an hotel and the next morning was found dead in bed from an over-dose of morphia. In this connection I had a curious experience a few years later, when I happened to stay a night at the hotel where this death had taken place. I was kept awake in the night by continual noises as if a lift were going up and down by the side of the room. After listening to the noise for most of the night and examining all the walls of the room with no result, I came to the conclusion that I was sleeping over a stable and that the noise was caused by horses dragging up the chains of their headstalls and then allowing the weights to fall down. This was the correct explanation. The next morning I went to the girl in the hotel office and said to her, "Why did you put me in Dr. X's room last night? His ghost kept me awake all night." She looked quite alarmed and evidently thought my question showed some uncanny knowledge. It was quite right; I had been put to sleep in that room.

Another excellent House-Surgeon, also from one of the leading Hospitals, was found by the old Matron one night in a very compromising situation with one of the Nurses. Of course both he and the Nurse were immediately discharged. One of my colleagues wanted me to refuse to give a testimonial to this man, but I gave it. He was a very capable officer and had fulfilled his surgical duties to my entire satisfaction, and that was all I stated in the testimonial. I still consider that I was right in doing this. I do not think it fair that a man should be eternally doomed for making a false step, even such a serious one, at the

182

outset of his career. His discharge was probably a good lesson for himself and for all the rest. As a matter of fact he did very well in his later career.

One of the best House-Surgeons we ever had was excellent at his work but very weak and flabby physically and he took no exercise. I used to discuss all sorts of topics with him; amongst them was suicide, and we agreed that we could not understand how anybody, and a medical man in particular, could destroy himself in such revolting ways as throat-cutting, etc. when there were obvious clean and easy methods at hand. When he left us he went on a voyage as a ship's surgeon and during this voyage he committed suicide by stabbing himself with a pen-knife in ten or twelve different places. I believe his mother was insane.

One of our House-Surgeons was a terrible cocainer. I have known him get up in the middle of dinner and go out of the room to take cocaine. I think he must have had a remarkable inside. He came to supper at my house one Sunday evening and there happened to be some stewed cherries on the table. I saw one of my boys looking very excitedly at the House-Surgeon's plate and it was only by frowning at him that I could keep him quiet. Afterwards the boy said to me, "Father, I had only one helping of cherries and there were sixty stones on my plate; the doctor had two helpings and did not leave a single stone." He was an exceptionally clever man, but the cocaine ruined him in the end. After he left us he got an appointment on the Gold Coast, and some of his acquaintances hoped and believed he would never come back. I said, "Don't you make any mistake; he is not the kind of man to die of yellow fever; he'll come back all right." He got the fever and a cablegram was sent to London, "The condition of Dr. X. is desperate; have called in the carpenter" (to make his coffin). Yet he came back after all, though I believe he eventually died in an asylum.

The stories of these unfortunate men should help us to realise that we are all human. The early part of the medical career is particularly trying to some young men, and many of those who fail to make good are more deserving of pity than of censure.

CHAPTER XXV

MATRONS AND NURSES

Matrons at Hospital. Gold medallist. Mortuary Chapel. Operating theatre. Linen Guild. Seventeen years. Presentation and tribute. War years. Present Matron. Training of Nurses. Nurses' League. Results. Gratitude. Respect for Nurses. Suggestions from Nurses.

My long experience of Matrons proves to me that The Kidderminster Hospital has been singularly fortunate in being able to secure the services of some exceptionally capable Matrons and to retain them for long periods.

The Matron when I joined the Staff was a very worthy old lady, but she had no idea of nursing or of surgery. However, she was a good house-keeper and she certainly had the interests of the hospital at heart.

Some years later a Matron was appointed who had previously won the gold medal at St. Bartholomew's Hospital. It was she who began the training of the nurses and put the nursing system on a proper basis, and she was very largely responsible for the exalted position our hospital came to hold among provincial hospitals. She was always on the alert to suggest and support anything that would improve the hospital and be of benefit to the patients. The mortuary chapel was largely the result of her initiative, she was very helpful in connection with the building of the operating theatre, which was opened in 1903, and she instituted the Ladies' Linen Guild, which is managed by a Committee of its own and undertakes to provide all the linen required by the hospital. She resigned in 1910 after seventeen years of excellent work. The following is an extract from the speech I made when a presentation was made to her:-

"I am pleased to have an opportunity to speak for the Staff and on their behalf to bear testimony to the good work that our Matron has accomplished during the past seventeen years; we are delighted to join in this presentation, which is a practical expression of our appreciation. I well remember her appointment. She came with a reputation, having obtained a gold medal at one of the leading hospitals in the kingdom. It was natural that much was expected from her and we can now confidently say that she has not only fulfilled but exceeded our expectations.

"Surgery in those days was in a transition stage and had it not been for the progress in nursing which has been such a conspicuous feature of her reign we could not have attained the position we now hold. Her work throughout has been marked by thoroughness; every detail has been attended to, regardless of the personal strain entailed, and all difficulties, however great, have been surmounted. The moral tone of the hospital has been kept at the highest level, while the welfare of the patients has always been placed in the forefront. The comfort of distressed relatives has received a consideration that can be bestowed only by one possessed of a kindly Christian spirit.

"We can all testify to these good qualities and our opinion of her is an expert one. The public may make mistakes, but the true estimate of one's worth is to be found amongst our fellow workers. She is one of the best Matrons who ever presided over a public institution."

She was succeeded by another great Matron, who was her own nominee, and who still further enhanced the reputation of the hospital. She was a most excellent Matron, a wonderful disciplinarian, and she attracted the very best type of nurse. During the war period she acted not only as Matron, but also as House-Surgeon. She had constantly to administer anaesthetics for me. She was often left in charge of from twelve to twenty serious cases upon whom operations had been performed during the day, and I can honestly put it on record that not once during those five years did she summon me up to the hospital unnecessarily and not once did she fail to summon me when it was necessary. That was a great achievement.

186

I have a profound admiration for her most valuable work, her skill, her kindness, and her self-sacrificing devotion to the hospital and the patients. The hospital is fortunate in retaining her services, for she still holds the position of Matron, and has done so for twenty-two years in all, with an interval of a few years in retirement. She also has carried on the training of nurses with conspicuous success, as is evidenced by the fact that since 1922 the hospital has been recognised as a First Class Training School for Nurses. She instituted the Nurses' League (of which more hereafter) in 1930 and its success testifies to the loyalty of the nurses to their training school.

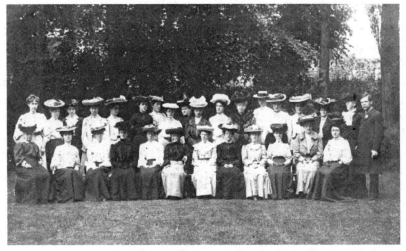

Lionel and his class of nurses ~1901

Many of the nurses trained here have done well later and some have attained high positions in the nursing profession. One is now a Matron in Canada. Another has become well known through her organisation of a successful system of making appointments for out-patients to see the members of the honorary staff of a hospital and so obviate the waiting that is sometimes such a disadvantage. She introduced this system in a hospital in the north of England and was afterwards invited to go to London and explain the system at a meeting there.

The following personal tribute goes to show that the training received at this hospital has borne good fruit and that the nurses themselves are not unmindful of the gratitude they owe for the care and skill displayed

187

in preparing them for their professional work. It is an extract from a letter received by one of our former nurses from a colleague, who also trained here and who was then working in Canada:-

"If you ever see Matron please tell her from me that I thank Mr. Stretton and herself from the bottom of my heart for the training I received at the Kidderminster Hospital. Also that I have never forgotten Mr. Stretton's parting speech, never to forget where we were trained and never to bring disgrace on our training school. I do not say this boastfully, but I am considered the best nurse who has been in this town."

Even when I was a medical student I realised that there was a great deal to be learnt from the Sisters and nurses in the hospital wards and I took every advantage of this. I hope I invariably treated them with due respect; I always felt it unwise to joke with them or be on too familiar terms with them. I am very angry with men who do not show them proper respect. It is absurd for a medical student or a doctor to try to make out that he knows everything and the nurses know nothing; there are many occasions when they know better than he does. Here is an instance of this.

Many years ago the Matron at the hospital telephoned down to me one night, "I feel very unhappy about one of your patients." "What is the matter?" I asked. "I feel sure he has tetanus," was her reply. "Well, what about the House-Surgeon?" "I dare not tell him; he would only be rude to me, yet I am quite sure I am right," she said. "Well," I replied, "I'll tell you what I will do. I am going out and I will look in at the hospital by accident." I did this and found the Matron was quite right. The man had got tetanus and the House-Surgeon did not know it, and if she had told him he would probably have been rude to her. It was a difficult position for the Matron.

I maintain that a man, and especially a young man, ought to be only too grateful for any suggestions and any help he can get from the nursing staff. After all, they are qualified people and they have often had a vast amount of experience. Fortunately nowadays most men do look at it in this light and are grateful for any suggestions the nurses can make.

188

CHAPTER XXVI

INAUGURATION OF THE HOSPITAL NURSES' LEAGUE

Members of Nurses' League. Welcome by Matron. Three Matrons. "Father."
Objects of League. Badge. Nursing profession. Conditions of work. Pension.
Examinations. Matrons. Loyalty.

The Nurses' League of The Kidderminster and District General Hospital was inaugurated at a meeting held in the Nurses' Home on the 29th October, 1930. Those eligible as members of the League are: (1) Nurses trained at the Hospital; (2) Nurses who have been trained elsewhere but have worked at this Hospital for at least one year. A considerable number of nurses who had been trained or had worked at the hospital attended the meeting and received a hearty welcome from the Matron, who spoke as follows:-

"I am very pleased to see you all and to be able to welcome those who trained and worked at this Hospital some years ago. We have Miss X. (a former Matron) with us, to whom we give a very hearty welcome, also Miss Y. (another former Matron) whom we are glad to see looking so bright and well after her serious illness.

"The work of Miss X., Miss Y. and myself covers a period of thirty-seven years, and it is to Miss X. that we owe the organisation of the proper training of nurses at this Hospital - a debt which can in no way be paid other than by loyalty and service to the dear old place.

"I thank you for making the effort to attend this meeting, for I know what very busy people you all are and how difficult it is to get away from your work. I hope that this meeting will keep us in touch with one another and also serve to keep up your interest in the Hospital and in all those who are training and have been trained in it. It has been a very great pleasure to me to know that so many are willing and anxious to join the League. I have received numbers of kind letters wishing us every success and it has been a great encouragement.

"It has been decided to have a badge in the shape of a shuttle, because this was thought to be appropriate for the Kidderminster Hospital, the shuttle playing so large a part in the industry of this carpet town."

The Matron then stated the objects of the League and referred to the Rules, which had been provisionally drawn up. After the President, other Officers, and members of the League had been elected the Matron asked me, as President and Senior Honorary Surgeon of the Hospital, to address the meeting, and I spoke as follows:

"Children, To justify myself in addressing you as children I must tell you that some years ago - it was one day during the war - I accidentally overheard part of a conversation between some of the nurses. The two words of that conversation that are indelibly imprinted on my mind are 'Father says.' I do not remember what Father said, but I do remember that I asked Matron about it and she told me that you all called me 'Father;' so I can call you 'Children.' I assure you I was very much gratified to know that you had given me a nickname that implied such affectionate esteem, and my gratification was increased by the knowledge that, as your Chief, it was my duty on occasions to reprimand some of you; but you were such a good lot of girls that those occasions were very rare. You may have thought it right and proper that a father should do the reprimanding.

"I suppose it is because you look upon me as a father that I have been asked to speak to you about the League that you are forming today. When Matron asked me to address you I was rather alarmed, because the word League is associated in my mind with a well-known League that has been instituted with the object of preventing quarrelling and fighting. I wondered why you had

190

become so bellicose as to need a League to enable you to keep the peace. I was relieved to find that the objects of your League are:-

> "1. To strengthen the bond of union between past and present members of the Nursing Staff;
>
> "2. To promote the honour, interest and usefulness of the Nursing Profession.

"The bond of union between you ought to be a very real one, and you should do all in your power to strengthen it. I feel sure that the formation of this League will assist you to do so. I am pleased to see that you have chosen a badge that can be worn as a brooch. Wear it always so that it can be seen, for wherever you are and whatever your position may be, there is always the possibility of a meeting with another woman who was trained at this Hospital. The badge will make you known to each other and will immediately constitute a bond of union, giving you interests in common and calling forth mutual attraction.

"You will both realise that you possess something in common, which you derived from The Kidderminster and District General Hospital and which is of inestimable value to you. What reminiscences you will indulge in! Pictures of the Hospital, descriptions of some of your colleagues, and your affectionate regard for your dear old Matron. I dare not suggest a nickname for her, but I have no doubt you have given her one.

"The other object of your League is to promote the honour, the interest, and the usefulness of the Nursing Profession.

"Amongst many other valuable lessons, you have learnt here what a power for good the Nursing Profession possesses. Most of you are aware of the high opinion I hold of your profession. Some of you may have read reports of speeches I have delivered, and one of them in which I stated that motherhood is the highest office that a woman can hold. I mention this today because I wish to say that the office of nurse follows it closely. I feel very strongly that everything that is possible should be done to promote the

191

honour, the interest and the usefulness of your profession. Individuals can do something, but a united body has much more influence. It has often been said that union is strength, and there is no doubt that union is necessary for the protection of the average nurse. The altruism of your profession has been exploited to such an extent that it is time to call a halt. Nurses have a right to demand fair conditions of labour and of pay. You should have regular hours of work and of rest; you should be properly housed and fed; you should have adequate recreation and holidays; you should be safeguarded against illness and accident and provided with compensation if you fall a victim to them; and you should be assured of a pension when you are no longer able to continue your work.

"Regular hours of work and rest are arranged so far as possible in hospitals, but in times of stress it may be necessary to increase your work, and no woman who is a nurse would object to this. But when the work slackens you should have extra leisure to make up for your extra work. Nurses who undertake private work may have twenty-four hours of continuous work at times, but they should not be expected to go on doing the work of two nurses in order to save expense to those who employ them.

"The demand for adequate housing for nurses is so strong that many hospitals are finding it necessary to provide extra accommodation, and we at the present time are building a new wing to our Nurses' Home, to contain thirty separate bedrooms. Private nurses should insist on having a separate room to sleep in.

"The most important provision is an adequate pension. We have started a Pensions Scheme here, but in my opinion a pension of £1 a week is not enough; it should be at least £2. Pensions should not be confined to hospital nurses. All nurses should have them. Half a guinea a week, or even a guinea a week, added to the fees for a private nurse would not be a very serious addition and it would enable this provision to be made. No-one ought to grudge this extra payment for such a purpose. There is nothing more pitiable than to see a woman stranded in her old age when she has given the best years of her life to nursing her fellow-men. Some of these fellow-men are mean enough to express their ingratitude by saying, 'Well, I have paid her.' The debt that a man owes to those who attend him in his illnesses can never be paid in money. He remains under an obligation which he should be ever ready to acknowledge, and he should do all in his power to assist those who attended him should they require it. He should remember that they may have served him at the risk of damage to their own health, perhaps at the risk of their life. It is appalling to know that some nurses have lived in poverty until forced into poor-houses to die, or have ended their lives by suicide.

"On the other hand, it is gratifying to know that the services of some of them have been handsomely requited by those who are of a generous disposition. But you ought to be safeguarded. A matter of such importance should not be left to chance. You should not be at the mercy of the disposition of those who employ you.

"You may call me an idealist and you may think that my ideas are impossible of attainment. I grant that it may take some time to effect such reforms, but I feel confident that they are bound to come, and they will come more quickly if you combine to make your demands. Remember that it is not only for your own good but it is for the good of your fellow-men, and it is in the interests of your country that the nursing profession should be recruited from the best material and that it should be kept in the highest state of efficiency. This cannot be accomplished unless the conditions under which you work are brought up to the level that I have indicated.

"The honour of your profession is in your hands. You must do your part and do it well. Some women are born nurses, and most women can attain proficiency if they work hard and put their hearts into their work. In these days of State examinations some of you have to suffer disappointments, but you should not be discouraged. Some of the best nurses may fail in an examination, and I know of no system that could make an examination a true indication of capability. I feel strongly that in all examinations - for whatever purpose - a report from the training school should be received and taken into account. It might prevent some very wrong decisions both ways. Put this forward at your League meeting and send it as a united suggestion. It might receive consideration and perhaps within the next fifty years it might be acted upon.

"Whatever your future may be you should never forget what you owe to your training school, and especially to the Matrons who have guided you through your training. I am sure you will all wish me to say how very fortunate The Kidderminster and District General Hospital has been in securing the services of such excellent Matrons. It was one of them who initiated the training of nurses here, and another has instituted the Nurses' League that we are inaugurating to-day.

"We are delighted to have Miss X. with us. She added lustre to the office of Matron of this Hospital, and it is well maintained today. We are delighted too to have Miss Y. with us and we are pleased to see her looking so well after the serious illness that deprived us of her valued services.

"Never forget your Matrons. Never forget your Hospital. Think of its glorious traditions; remember that its honour lies largely in your hands, for your work and your conduct both now and in the future will be powerful factors in determining its reputation. To show yourselves worthy of your training is a duty you owe to yourselves, a duty you owe to your Hospital, and, above all, a duty you owe to your noble profession."

CHAPTER XXVII

SOME PROFESSIONAL EXPERIENCES

Nurses' League, 1936. Paré's dictum and my addition. Missing swabs. Fainting in theatre. Assistants. Administration of anaesthetics. A critical operation. Drunkenness and drugs. Portable operation table. Early Nursing Homes. Quick work. Preparation of patients. A night's experience. A drunken cook. Simple methods. Surgical cleanliness. Importance of nurses.

The Matron asked me to give an address at the annual meeting of the Nurses' League in November, 1936. I felt sure that an account of some of my professional experiences would be of interest to the nurses and I therefore gave them the following address. Some passages are omitted from this chapter, either because the substance of them has appeared in earlier chapters or because they are hardly suitable for inclusion in a book intended for the general public.

"When the Matron asked me to address you this afternoon I welcomed the opportunity to express my admiration of the nursing profession. The great French surgeon Paré said: 'I operate on the patients, but God cures them.' To my mind he might have added that God's most important instrument in curing the patient is the nurse. An operation is a team job, in which the operator takes the lead; but the assistant and the anaesthetist are important, and so are the nurses.

"Only last month I was forcibly reminded of the value of the nurses. After an abdominal operation I had nearly finished suturing the peritoneum when Sister told me that a swab was missing. I relaxed my suture and found the swab, which I extracted. I said, 'Good girl' I may in the first instance have said 'Damn!' It is one of the bad habits one acquires. But there is more

195

than one way of saying 'Damn!' and I think you will all agree that I never say it excitedly or maliciously. I remember on another occasion when I had sutured the skin I was obliged to open up the abdomen to look for a missing swab, and while I was looking for it I heard the welcome news that it had been found. I did not swear; I complimented my nurses on having the courage to say that it was lost until they had found it. On another occasion when I turned to take a swab from the nurse who was holding them I noticed that she was about to collapse. I said, 'Lay her on the floor and pull her outside.'

"It is no disgrace to feel faint in the theatre. Even surgeons may succumb. Some years ago I was operating on a thyroid. The anaesthetic was being administered by an experienced House-Surgeon who had previously served a year as House-Surgeon in one of the leading hospitals. As often happens, there was a gush of blood from a vein. I heard the House-Surgeon say, 'Very bad,' and I looked up at him just in time to tell the nurses to lay him down on the floor and drag him out. I had only the Sister helping me, so I asked one of the nurses to carry on with the anaesthetic, under my direction, and I completed the operation without mishap.

"One week-end I had a distinguished surgeon from London staying with me. In the evening I received an urgent summons to the hospital to perform an abdominal operation. The surgeon asked if he might accompany me, and when we arrived in the theatre he asked if he might assist me. After a minute or two I looked up and saw at once that he was about to collapse. I said, 'Lay him on the floor and drag him out!' He was a game man, for when he thought he had recovered he came back, but only to collapse again and again be dragged out.

"Assistants are important, and it adds very much to the comfort of the surgeon if his assistant is familiar with his technique. In the olden days it was the privilege of the assistant surgeon to help his chief at operations. Sir William Lawrence is reported to have said that his junior was such an excellent assistant that he ought never to be made a surgeon. Some of the Sisters and nurses make excellent assistants, and I often think of a doctor who said to me,

'If ever I have to undergo an operation you must do it, Sister must help you, and Matron must give me the anaesthetic.'

"In my early days it was the custom for the anaesthetic to be administered by the doctor in attendance, who seldom knew anything about it, and as a result I had some anxious experiences. On one occasion I was sent for into the country to perform an abdominal operation. As instructed by the doctor in attendance, I went by train and took the Theatre Sister with me. At the station we were met by the doctor in a small pony-trap, in which with great difficulty we packed the Sister and the paraphernalia. I was instructed to walk along the road until I reached a white gate; I was then to cross a field until I came to a river where there was a boat, and I was to wait for a man to row me over.

"When we eventually arrived we found a very stout old lady with a strangulated umbilical hernia. It was then about 3.30 on a winter afternoon. The doctor volunteered to give the anaesthetic while Sister and I did the sterilising and preparation of instruments and dressings. When we had been at this for about half an hour I asked Sister to see how the patient was getting on. She returned to tell me that the doctor would never get her under, so I went and had a look. The doctor was using a weird and wonderful inhaler with a pair of bellows, which he was constantly squeezing. Every minute or two he would say, 'Hold your hand up, my dear,' and up came the hand with unfailing regularity. It was then getting dusk, so I had to arrange for lamps and candles and get the kitchen table up to act as an operating table, and still the patient's hand went up!

"Eventually I had to put her under the anaesthetic myself and trust to the doctor to keep it up, which of course he did not do. There was Sister on one side, with a great paraffin lamp standing on the table by the side of the patient, and myself on the other. When I opened the abdomen I found about three feet of gangrenous intestine, which I had to excise.

"In those days we used a Murphy's button in such operations. How Sister, and I escaped being burnt to death I do not know, but

197

we got through. I then asked the doctor when the last train went back. He replied, 'Oh, it has gone; there isn't another today.'

"I had to send a man on foot four miles to telegraph for my Brougham, and when it arrived, at about 8 o'clock, the horses had to be rested for a couple of hours before they could face the return journey of 20 miles. Sister and I were quite happy and we reached home in the small hours of the next morning. I had told the doctor how to treat the patient and asked him not to give her any morphia. He demurred and said she was four miles away from him and he could not be running over to see her often. [7]

"Five days later he wrote and told me that the old lady had died comatose, and that the result of the operation was perfect; he returned my Murphy's button. I expect her coma was due to morphia. I was very fortunate in having such an excellent nurse to help me. Alas! She ended her life by throwing herself out of a window; she was found dead on the pavement below. Probably cocaine. Suicide, drunkenness, and drugs are the sad sides of the careers of nurses and doctors, and I have had far too many experiences connected with them.

"It was after that operation that I invented a portable operation table that would wrap up neatly. Previous ones rolled up like an old market woman's umbrella; mine rolls up like a Mayfair umbrella. Since the advent of the Nursing Home this has become unnecessary. I remember the first Nursing Home I visited. A lady patient of my father had a breast removed. The operation was performed on a four-poster bedstead, and I had to lie by the side of the patient to administer the anaesthetic. That was at a Nursing Home in a large town in the midlands. The nurses had a difficult task and it is much to their credit that the wound healed without any complication.

"Nursing Homes now are much more satisfactory; we have little difficulty in persuading most patients to enter them and in

---

[7] See Addendum 2.2

these days of motor ambulances it is easy to transport them. I have brought many a patient to my Nursing Home in my own car. A typical example is that of a lady who was in labour. I brought her fifteen miles in my car and she was comfortably in bed with her baby, after a Caesarean section, within an hour and a half of starting from her home. She told me she had a most comfortable journey, and the nurse was well pleased. But wasn't the doctor horrified at the risk! On another occasion I brought the senior physician from a town about 40 miles away, and I had him in bed, after removing his prostate, in less than two hours from the time we left his home.

"These two examples show that the extensive preparation of patients undertaken in many cases is not a necessity. We are proud of the fact that the sterilisation of the skin with tincture of iodine was discovered in this hospital[8], and we know that previous scrubbing and washing is not only unnecessary but harmful. We also know that aperients and enemas are not essential; they often do harm.

"I have been obliged to dismiss several nurses because of their drunkenness or drug-taking, and of course it is impossible to employ or recommend them again. They might cause injury or death. Even a domestic servant may endanger life. I remember an experience I had one winter night when the snow was on the ground. I had been attending a lady in her confinement and did not get back to bed until after midnight. An hour later my cook, who answered the night bell, called me to say that the lady I had attended was suffering from severe haemorrhage. I hurried up and in order to save time I trotted up to her house, about a mile away, as it was quicker than ordering out my carriage.

"When I arrived at the house all was in darkness. After I had rung the bell vigorously several times the old nurse midwife put her head out of a window and said, 'Why, Mr. Stretton, what ever

---

[8] See Addendum 1

is the matter?' I told her she had sent for me because of haemorrhage. 'O no,' she said, 'I have not sent for you.' I hurried back home, wondering who the patient was that was suffering from bleeding, and I bethought me that it must be an old gentleman who was subject to attacks of haemoptysis. He lived in a large house three or four miles away and it was his custom to send one of his footmen on a bicycle to summon me when necessary. I woke up the cook and asked if the name was not the name of this gentleman and if the messenger was a man on a bicycle; the name was somewhat similar. 'O yes,' she said, 'that was the name and a man did come on a bicycle.' I hurried out my carriage and rushed off.

"On arrival at the house I rang the bell. The butler's head came out of a window and he said, 'Why, Mr. Stretton, what ever is the matter?' I told him that his master was bleeding and had sent for me. 'No,' he said, 'the master is quite comfortable.' So I drove quickly home. While I was questioning my cook again my coachman shouted up, 'It's all right, Sir. The gentlemen has come again.' The patient who needed my services lived a couple of miles in the opposite direction and she and her relatives had been through a very anxious time. I had suffered too, and the patient might have lost her life.

"The next day I found that the cause of all this trouble was my whisky, which my cook had been drinking. She was an excellent cook, she had no relations, and I felt that if I turned her out she might have to go to the work-house. So I made her sign a pledge for twelve months and promised her a character if she kept it. To my surprise she did keep it, and she then went to an acquaintance of mine, to whom I told the story. He was very pleased with her cooking, but alas, she relapsed, and he was obliged to send her away.

"You all know that I adopt very simple methods. I use few instruments and I operate quickly, but never in a hurry. I do not wear any masks or hats; I gave them up more than thirty years ago, because I found that they caused sweating, which is a far greater danger than any benefit they can give. I have lived through many forms of surgical ritualism, including the carbolic spray, and I have often quoted the words of one of the greatest surgeons I have ever known - Sir William Savory, who gave the address on surgery at the meeting of the British Medical Association held in Cork about 1879. In his peroration he said: 'Gentlemen, when the history of surgery comes to be written, you will find that it is not a question of the steam spray, it is not a question of carbolic acid, it is a question of surgical cleanliness! And he was right.

"To you nurses I say: the cure of a patient is not only a question of the surgeon; it is not only a question of his assistants, but it is largely a question of the nurses."

202

CHAPTER XXVIII

SOME GREAT MEN IN THE PROFESSION

Greatness. Personality. Test of time. Hippocrates. William Harvey. John Hunter. One hundred years. W.G. Grace. Joseph Lister. Louis Pasteur. Robert Koch. Rudolf Virchow. Ambroise Paré. Charles Hastings and the British Medical Association. William Gull. John Abernethy. Percivall Pott. Spencer Wells. James Paget. Luther Holden. Henry Thompson. Andrew Clarke. Matthews Duncan. James Young Simpson and chloroform. James Syme. William Savory. Anaesthetists. William Macewen. Lauder Brunton. William Jenner and others.

As President of the Kidderminster Medical Society for many years, it has been my duty to give an address at the annual dinner of the Society. Such an after-dinner speech is not necessarily of a scientific character, but its subject usually has some connection with our profession. This chapter is taken from the address I gave in 1928.

"Some are born great, some achieve greatness, and some have greatness thrust upon them." Most people are familiar with this quotation. Like many other quotations, it contains some truth, but I am not prepared to accept it as entirely true. No man can achieve greatness unless he is born with the necessary germ-plasm. He may have a great position thrust upon him, but that will not make him a great man.

There are varieties of greatness, which it is difficult, if not impossible, to define. A man may be great as compared with his contemporaries but not great in the history of the world. A man may have a great personality, a quality that is likely to die with him, because a personality cannot be portrayed with exactitude. A man will be known in the future by the work he has accomplished, and one of the best measures of his greatness will be the length of time he is remembered after his death and the value that will be attributed to his work by future generations.

In my own profession the name of Hippocrates is still remembered, after more than two thousand years, and I cannot imagine that such names as William Harvey and John Hunter will ever be forgotten. But the majority of so-called great men are only men of prominence during the period in which they live, and most of them will be forgotten ten years after their death. Very few will be remembered one hundred years after their death. I believe that only three of the men I have known will be remembered one hundred years after their death; these three are Joseph Lister, Robert Koch, and W.G. Grace. I was at St. Bartholomew's Hospital with W.G. Grace and I need hardly specify what he will be remembered for. Although the number of centuries he made at cricket has since been eclipsed it must be remembered that Grace was an amateur and played under more difficult conditions than were enjoyed by later players of eminence, and his record therefore stands. I think it may stand for centuries.

I had the advantage of seeing Lister operate at King's College Hospital; he was dressed in a black mackintosh and enveloped in his carbolic spray. He was a kindly, mild-spoken man. He had not a great personality but he immortalised himself by revolutionising surgery and his name, in conjunction with that of Louis Pasteur, will probably live for ever.

As already described, I saw Koch in Berlin at the time of the great rush there to study his tuberculin. He was a very shy, retiring man, but his discovery of the tubercle bacillus has made his name immortal. It is interesting to know that it was while he was engaged in general practice that he conducted the experiments that led to his discovery of the tubercle bacillus. The animals he used for his experiments[9] were kept in his stable. Had he lived in this country his work could not have been done, because some of our laws are passed to satisfy agitators, in defiance of scientific opinion and without regard for the welfare of the human race.

----

[9] See Addendum 5.5

I have also referred to my meeting with Virchow in Berlin. He was a great little man of a kind and courteous disposition. He devoted a whole morning to showing my colleague and myself round his department at the Charité Hospital.

Everyone in my profession knows something about the great men who have lived during the last few centuries. Ambroise Paré, the French surgeon, who re-introduced the use of the ligature, was wont to say, "I operate upon the patients, but God cures them." We may say God, or Nature, or any other name, but there is no doubt that the result of an operation does not depend entirely upon the surgeon. A great deal of the success depends upon him and his assistants, including the nurses; but there is an influence for good or ill that is not under his control. Most surgeons have seen patients die when they felt sure they would recover, and have seen patients recover when they felt sure they would die. There is some intangible and unseen influence at work that decides the result. And where would plastic surgery be without the co-operation of Nature?

I have already alluded to William Harvey and John Hunter, whose names are as household words to members of the profession.

Passing on to a period nearer the present time, I have heard my father speak of Charles Hastings, of Worcester. He it was who founded the British Medical Association, and this should ensure the remembrance of his name for all time.

William Gull will be remembered for his work on typhoid fever and his attendance upon the Prince of Wales (afterwards King Edward VII) when he was ill with that disease. He once came down here to meet my father in consultation and very much surprised him by refusing to accept any hospitality. He explained that it was his custom to carry a pocketful of raisins for his refreshment when necessary. I am not sure if it was he who refused lunch at a patient's house, because he considered that he was looked upon as an oracle and that if he had a meal with the family it would lessen his prestige. When he died he left the largest fortune that has been left by any member of the medical profession; I believe it was £350,000.

John Abernethy, the founder of the Medical School at St. Bartholomew's Hospital, was an able teacher and did some original work in surgery. I believe he was a great personality. Many amusing stories are told of him; for instance, how he met a talkative woman in Newgate Street, instructed her to shut her eyes tight and put out her tongue, and how he then got away from her by running round the next corner.

Percival Pott was a surgeon at St. Bartholomew's Hospital and a great teacher of surgery. The terms 'Pott's fracture,' 'Pott's disease of the spine,' and 'Pott's puffy swelling' are still in use and may perpetuate his name.

I have been fortunate in being intimately acquainted with many of the prominent men in the profession during my lifetime. Spencer Wells was a surgeon in the Crimea during the War and my father was associated with him there. He will be remembered for some years because of his courage in performing ovariotomies in spite of great opposition. I remember seeing him perform one of these operations in Kidderminster. So far as I can remember there were none of the aseptic precautions that we are used to in these days, but the patient did well.

James Paget was President of the Royal College of Surgeons, a member of the surgical staff at St. Bartholomew's, and surgeon to Queen Victoria. He should be remembered for his clinical and microscopical work on tumours. He was a delightful character, as were all the members of his family. I used to go to his house sometimes on Sundays, when there was a happy family gathering. Sometimes we had tea in the nursery with the old Nanna. We waited on ourselves at supper and afterwards had songs in the drawing-room.

I have already referred to Luther Holden in connection with my training at St. Bartholomew's. His book on osteology is well known. He was a typical English gentleman and was very much beloved by the students. He was supposed to be a very lenient examiner. When a student went into the room trembling Holden would take him by the arm and lead him up to a microscope: "Now, young man, look through that microscope and you will see some blood." The boy would look through the microscope, smile up at Holden and say, "Yes, Sir, it is blood." Holden would say, "Quite right. Now go and look down that next microscope and tell me what you see there." And woe betide him if he was wrong. Holden had put him at his ease and gained his confidence, and I believe he plucked more men than any other examiner. That was his method, and a very correct method.

Henry Thompson was a good surgeon and specially noted as a lithotomist. He performed lithotomy on Leopold I, King of the Belgians and on the Emperor Napoleon III. He came to Kidderminster on two occasions to operate and I can hear him now explaining to me the most important points about the operation. He performed his operations in the most artistic manner.

Andrew Clarke was a Scotsman and had a great personality. He told me how in his early days he was sent abroad to die of phthisis; but he recovered, came back to London and became one the most successful physicians there. He left a quarter of a million of money when he died, all of which he had made himself. He told me once that he was making an income of £20,000 a year, and £10,000 of it in his consulting room, where he saw large numbers of patients. He told me also that he owed his success in a large measure to a chance call to a gentleman who was fainting in the street, and who was none other than Mr. Gladstone. Many interesting stories are told about Clarke. On one occasion he was summoned to the south of France to see a patient, an old lady, for a fee of 500 guineas. He replied that he was unable to go. When another telegram was sent to him offering him 1,000 guineas he was still unable to go; and the telegrams continued to arrive, with the fee rising by a thousand guineas a time until it reached 5,000 guineas. Clarke then went. When he was offered his cheque for 5,000 guineas he refused it, saying that his fee was 500 guineas, and that the reason he had not gone when first summoned was that he was unable to go; and he resolutely refused to take more than the 500 guineas. It was very much to his credit, and it was to the old lady's credit that she asked him to decide to what charity the remainder of, the money should be given.

Matthews Duncan had come to St. Bartholomew's Hospital when I went there. He was a great teacher of gynaecology and a very kindly man. He told me the story about chloroform. James Syme and Matthews Duncan were dining with James Young Simpson at his house one night. When the ladies had left the table these three men decided to test the anaesthetic properties of chloroform, which Simpson had discovered. Shortly afterwards they were all found unconscious under the dining-table. Syme was recognised as a great authority on surgery and Simpson probably immortalised himself by his discovery of chloroform anaesthesia. I did not know either of them.

I consider that William Savory was the greatest personality that I have ever known in the profession. In addition to being a good surgeon he was a great orator. When he felt disagreement or contempt he never hesitated to express them and he was noted for his cutting remarks, though I feel sure he did not mean to be unkind. On one occasion when he was operating at St. Bartholomew's Hospital he sent for me to give an anaesthetic to a beery drayman. There were twenty or thirty students round the bed, and in vain I tried to get the man under ether. I turned to Mr. Savory and I said, "I cannot get him under the ether, Sir. Do you mind if I give him some chloroform?" He looked at me with his sardonic smile and said, "I sent for you to anaesthetise the patient, Stretton." His remark called forth roars of laughter from the students. I do not think he meant it unkindly. There had been trouble in the hospital some years before because one of the surgeons ordered the anaesthetist to give ether to a patient; he gave it under protest, and the patient died. After that an order was issued that the surgeons were not to interfere with the anaesthetists, which is quite right.

It is given to very few surgeons to live more than seventy years and still be on the active staff of their hospitals, as William Macewen was. I never knew him but I always recognised that he was a great surgeon. He did much original work on brain and mastoid surgery and on catgut ligatures. He discovered the method of preparing these ligatures so that they would last for varying periods.

Lauder Brunton was an excellent physician and did a great deal of work on the heart and blood pressure. He it was who advocated the use of strychnine, which is still used as a heart stimulant.

I have referred to only a few of the eminent men I have known. Among others were: William Jenner, Thomas Smith, Richard Douglas Powell, Henry Butlin, Malcolm Morris, Samuel Gee, and Dyce Duckworth. All were distinguished in various ways, yet it is doubtful whether any of them, except the few outstanding ones I have specially mentioned, will be remembered after one hundred years.

CHAPTER XXIX

THE SURGEON AND HIS WORK

Definite views on surgery. Surgeons born not made. Training, general and special. Apprenticeship. Incompetent operators. Diploma for operators. Minor operations. Surgery and general practice. Team work. Nurses. Attributes of surgeon. Health. Physique. Personal characteristics. Special senses. Love of surgery. Capacity. Postponement of operations. Rapid decision and prompt action. Mistakes. Faulty teaching. Thoroughness. Observation. Promptness. Multiple operations. Courage. Inoperable. Two cases. Judicial mind. Law Courts. Notes of cases. Teaching. Rapidity. Artistry. Surgical temperament. Coolness. Self-control. Limited communities. Relations.

An experience of more than fifty-six years, constant observation, and thought, have given me very definite views on surgery in general and the attributes of a surgeon in particular. Some of these views I have already alluded to, but in this chapter I propose to set them forth more fully, illustrating some of the points by experiences of my own.

It is probably correct to say that surgeons, like poets, are born, not made. But even a born surgeon must be trained before he can become competent, and the training cannot be too general or too thorough. Medicine must be studied as well as surgery, because the border-line between them is not clearly defined. If a man is to attain clinical acumen and diagnostic skill he must have knowledge of all branches or the profession.

I was fortunate in being apprenticed. As I have already indicated, that early training has been one of my most useful possessions. It gave me a knowledge of minor ailments and of many practical points; even such details as the methods of cleaning instruments and mixing lotions are items of knowledge not to be despised. It is said that such knowledge can be more profitably acquired by a man after he is qualified. My experience of House-Surgeons and Assistants does not bear out this assertion. Some of these young men have made excellent officers, but many of them despised detail and suffered so severely from the condition known as "swelled head" that it was difficult to teach them.

I do not deny that surgeons of a mediocre type can be made; but such men will never become distinguished, because they do not possess the necessary qualities. One of the saddest aspects of surgery today is the fact that any man who possesses a registered qualification in medicine or surgery is entitled to perform any operation he is willing to undertake. Fortunately most men refuse to accept such a responsibility, yet many do undertake operations that they are incompetent to perform. The results are appalling to contemplate. If I were to give illustrations of cases that I have seen or that have been described to me they would probably not be believed. Attention has been drawn to this question by several surgeons, but so far no attempt has been made to protect the public from incompetent operators and so prevent the surgical tragedies that are occurring daily.

The man who performs only occasional operations would be wiser not to perform one at all. Operative surgery demands constant practice. In order to obtain this a surgeon must have thirty or forty beds at his disposal in a properly equipped hospital. Cottage hospitals should draft their operation cases to larger institutions. This should not be difficult with the transport facilities available at the present time. For exceptional cases where it is undesirable to move the patient the services of a skilled operator can always be procured.

Operating surgeons should be specially trained and when competent they should be given a diploma entitling them to operate. A course of lessons in operative surgery on the cadaver is no guarantee that a man is a competent operating surgeon. Even his possession of the coveted F.R.C.S. Eng. is no proof of his ability to perform surgical operations. The training should be practical as well as theoretical. A candidate for an ordinary qualification is obliged to produce evidence that he has attended a certain number of confinements. In like manner a candidate for a diploma in operative surgery should be obliged to produce evidence that he has performed a certain number of major operations, of varied types, under the supervision of an experienced surgeon, before he is admitted for examination.

I would make it a penal offence for anyone to perform a major operation if he did not possess the qualification for operative surgery, unless the operation was performed under the supervision of an experienced operating surgeon, or unless he could prove that the services of a qualified operating surgeon were unobtainable and the case was an urgent one. Major operations would have to be defined and tabulated, and some specialist operators would be necessary, for instance, ophthalmic surgeons. I have no hesitation in stating that I consider it less dangerous to the public for a druggist to attend a case of pneumonia than for a general practitioner to undertake an abdominal section.

Even minor operations are best left in the hands of qualified operating surgeons; it would be better for the patient, more satisfactory to the relatives, and less worrying to the general practitioner. Sepsis may follow a circumcision and cause trouble and anxiety, and even danger to life. If a general practitioner has performed the operation the relations and friends of the patient are apt to say that such a complication would not have occurred if the operator had been a skilful surgeon; and such statements are not always incorrect. The removal of a uvula may be followed by a serious haemorrhage; tonsillectomy may cause death. Mistakes may be made, such as the amputation of a sound finger instead of a stiff one, to which I have already referred. The greater my experience, the more convinced I am that a general practitioner should decline all operative work, in the interests both of his patients and of himself.

It may seem curious that I should write this, for I developed my own surgery while I was carrying on an extensive general practice. This has proved to me that I should have been wiser if I had confined my work to surgery. Like many others, I was a victim of circumstances; I was obliged to assist my father in his practice to enable him to bring up his large family. Fortunately I was on the staff of a hospital that provided me with a sufficient number of beds, and the general practice allowed me time to carry on my surgical work. I soon found out, however, that general practice and surgery are not compatible. I cannot explain why this should be so, but I know that the general practice rapidly dwindled, and it was not because I refused to continue it.

Operative surgery is a team job and it is essential that a surgeon should be able to secure capable assistants. Unless a man is distinguished he will not be able to command the best assistance. The anaesthetist is of the first importance and it is generally possible to obtain the services of an expert, though in an emergency operation it may be necessary to be satisfied with an unpractised administrator. The assistant should be one who regularly fills this position. I prefer a trained nurse. A capable woman will soon learn a surgeon's methods and be able to anticipate his movements and his requirements. She must be a woman who can be trusted to do all the sterilising, to take charge of the instruments and prepare the sutures, ligatures, and dressings. In this respect a junior surgeon is handicapped, but he generally acts as assistant to a senior man, who will provide him with a team for such cases as come his way.

Many attributes are desirable in a surgeon, but it is seldom that they are all combined in one man; hence the limited supply of first-class surgeons. A surgeon should have good health, for a man cannot do good work if he is in ill health. The work of a surgeon is very trying and he is often exposed to risks. There may be an infection, which would easily kill a man in ill health; there may be loss of rest or exposure to bad weather, which he could not withstand. These risks can best be guarded against by living carefully and avoiding excesses of all kinds. A surgeon must be a man of strong physique, because he often has to perform duties requiring muscular strength. He should possess a skin that does not easily chafe or perspire, manual dexterity, and hands that are not large, that is, not above size 8. I am fortunate in having hands of different sizes, and as my left is the smaller, size 7¼, I find it advantageous to use it for exploration purposes. It is obvious that a 7¼ hand can enter a smaller opening than an 8 hand; this means a smaller incision and less suturing for closure. It is of great value to the surgeon to be ambidextrous and this faculty should be cultivated on all possible occasions.

A surgeon's tactile sensibility must be acute for both diagnostic and operative purposes; indeed, all the special senses should be acute, for all are of value. The trained eye will see many conditions that would escape

214

the notice of the untrained - conditions that may be of importance as aids to diagnosis or indications for treatment. A trained sense of smell will be able to recognise the distinctive odour of some diseases, for instance, carcinoma. Some diseases may be tasted; indeed they seem to affect one's tissues generally. An acute sense of taste will help in judging whether prescriptions have been accurately dispensed and in appraising the value of food, wines, and spirits. Acuteness of hearing is of value in auscultation, which should not be left entirely to the physician. It is a surgeon's duty to hear the foetal heart and to decide upon the presence or absence of fluid in the pleura or the pericardium. A trained hand in the abdomen will discover conditions which could not otherwise be ascertained without performing a more extensive incision and a prolonged operation.

A surgeon must have a great love of and a great capacity for his work. I do not agree that, because he loves it, it is play, as suggested by Tom Sawyer in the words: "Work consists of whatever a body is obliged to do and play consists of whatever a body is not obliged to do." No man can do operative surgery well unless he loves it. Dislike of the work is fatal, and indifference leads to careless and slovenly performances. The effort is mental as well as physical and at times it may be prolonged. Capacity is often put to a severe test; on many occasions I have stood for six hours on end at my operating table. No man can foretell how long or how difficult an operation may be. Once begun, it must be carried through to the end; there must be no delay. No competent surgeon would stop to consult books during an operation, nor would he rest and smoke a cigarette while considering what to do next, as may be done with impunity in other walks of life. When one operation has been completed others may have to be performed. There may be an emergency operation that cannot be delayed. A series of operations may have been arranged. It is true that some of them might be postponed, but from a humane point of view it is not right to subject a patient to a second preparation if it can be avoided. A surgeon ought to realise that an operation is a great ordeal to the majority of patients and he should do all in his power to lighten it, and especially should he guard against the repetition of the ordeal which would be caused by a postponement of the operation. It should be remembered also that some patients will not face it a second time. It may be that if a surgeon is tired he cannot do good work, and here comes in again the question of capacity. A surgeon should know his own limitations and, so far as possible, should not arrange to do more than is well within his powers. Then if an unforeseen case is thrust upon him he will be able to deal with it.

A surgeon must be a man of decision and he should ever keep before him the knowledge that upon his decision may depend the life of a human being. He must therefore do all in his power to improve his knowledge and his technique and to keep himself always ready and fit. He must not hesitate or procrastinate but always bear in mind the fact that large numbers of people die daily because the treatment is too late to save them. It is a tragedy for a patient in a hospital to die because an operation has been postponed, the so-called surgeon having been unable to make up his mind to perform it. If a surgeon thinks that an operation is necessary he will perform it, and he would rather perform twenty operations that prove to be unnecessary than omit to perform one the omission of which causes the death of the patient.

The decisions of a surgeon cannot always be as deliberate as those of a physician, and he often has to take immediate action based upon his decision. But though his decision has to be rapid it should be well considered, and this depends upon his training and his experience combined with surgical instinct, which is a thing inborn. A man who hesitates and alters his opinion is like a player at bridge who pulls out a card, puts it back, hesitates and then pulls out another, and so on, and he generally plays the wrong card in the end. Such a man will never make a surgeon. Having once made his decision the surgeon must not alter it, and he should not regret it or question the wisdom of it. He will not always be right; no-one is. If he makes a mistake he must not be discouraged; he should have a philosophic mind and realise that more can be learnt from mistakes than from successes. The best cricketer may fail to make a run, and the best surgeon will operate more skilfully at one time than at another and arrive at more accurate diagnoses. He is unlikely to do his best work when called up in the night - a fact which might with advantage be kept in mind by the profession and the public. If you wished a cricketer to score a century you would not arouse him from his slumbers to attempt the task.

216

There are mistakes that are pardonable and mistakes that are unpardonable. The latter ought never to occur in the practice of a surgeon. Such a mistake is the removal of a roll of great omentum in mistake for an appendix. Yet such an unpardonable blunder was, thus described in a clinical lecture on surgery:-

"One thing I am sure you will do, because we have all done it, is to take away a piece of omentum, and declare you have removed the appendix. In a fat subject you may find a piece of omentum, shaped like an appendix, which you will tie off and remove, quite satisfied that the patient will do very well; but in a couple of months, or less, he will come back with another attack of appendicitis. Then you will have to allow that some people must have more than one appendix. Really, it is a case of carelessness on your part, because what you removed had no lumen and no mucous membrane, only you never looked to see before the operation was completed. The knowledge that you are liable to these errors will be your best safeguard against falling into them."

I sometimes wonder whom the lecturer meant by "we." Such teaching is most dangerous for students.

As another instance of bad teaching for students I may quote a case of a youth who was admitted to hospital with a crushed forearm. The surgeon decided to amputate. After the operation he examined the mangled remains and remarked to the assembled students, "I believe I could have saved the arm."

Thoroughness is valuable in all walks of life, but it is particularly important in surgery. "Teach me to be more thorough has been my orison, and I have tried to inspire my assistants with this virtue. I have always kept before me, "Whatsoever thy hand findeth to do, do it with thy might," and I have amplified this by the word all - all thy might.

No man can be thorough in his work unless he is observant. It is easy to overlook important facts and conditions. A surgeon should lose no opportunity of increasing his powers of observation. Some advocate the habit of noticing and memorising the articles in a shop window; piecing together a jig-saw puzzle and playing bridge are both also helpful in this respect.

A man who is thorough will also be prompt. He will not put off until tomorrow what may be done today, because he does not know what demands tomorrow may make upon him. He will be punctual in keeping his appointments and have regard for the time of others as well as his own. He will attend to his correspondence daily, and he will always remember that prompt action may be the determining factor in saving life. Hours - even minutes - may be of importance.

Many errors are committed for want of thoroughness, and this is especially true in operative work. It is a calamity to remove some gall-stones and leave a gangrenous appendix to cause death. Yet, a surgeon may err in the opposite direction. To linger over an operation and make prolonged investigations may be wrong, especially in acute cases, but a rapid survey is always desirable. When multiple pathological changes are found demanding operation it is not always advisable to perform all the operations at the same time, though it may be necessary to do more than one. There is a limit to human endurance and it is not justifiable to increase the risk to life by a further operation unless it is probable that death will follow unless this is undertaken without delay. It is in such cases that courage is so essential to a surgeon.

If a surgeon is satisfied that an operation is a justifiable risk there should be no hesitation in performing it, provided that he has explained the risk to the patient and the relatives and obtained their consent to it. A man who refuses to undertake an operation for fear lest it should damage his statistics is not worthy of the name of surgeon. Some conditions are described as inoperable. What exactly the word inoperable is intended to convey I do not know. But I should like to stress the point that, provided that the patient and his friends consent to it, an operation may be not only justifiable but desirable in order to enable the sufferer to die more comfortably. I may quote two cases, out of many, to illustrate these points: 1. a man with a carcinoma of his right maxilla came to me. He was a bad subject for operation and the condition had been pronounced inoperable, but he was anxious to be rid of his fetid growth. I made a free removal of his right maxilla; he had no recurrence of the disease and lived for nearly twenty years afterwards. 2. a woman with a

218

fungating carcinoma of her right breast came and begged me to help her. The smell was horrible and she was in the greatest distress. I made a free removal of the mass, which operation gave her six months of comparatively comfortable existence; she ultimately died of an internal recurrence, with a minimum of discomfort. Her gratitude to me for having freed her from the growth was very great.

A judicial mind will enable a surgeon to examine signs and symptoms put before him and to draw conclusions from them. He must especially guard against any prejudice produced by a former diagnosis. This judicial mind will also be valuable when he is giving evidence in a Law Court. Cross-examination is an ordeal to some men and they sometimes make contradictory statements. Much of the adverse criticism advanced against the medical profession as expert witnesses is due more to their incompetence as witnesses than to any misrepresentation of facts. If questions can be answered by Yes or No it is wise to give these answers. If a question is not understood a full explanation should be demanded. The last part of the chapter on legal experiences illustrates this point.

A surgeon should have descriptive power and be able to make exact notes. To write down that a patient has a small tumour which he has noticed for a long time conveys nothing to the mind of a scientific man. Notes may be necessary when evidence has to be given in Court; they may need to be referred to when the writer is not available and when points of detail that appeared trivial at the time may be of value. Notes may indicate a tendency to haemorrhage or some other idiosyncrasy that may be guarded against. I do not suggest that it is necessary for a surgeon always to write his own notes, but it is his duty to see that they are accurately kept.

A surgeon must be able to explain conditions clearly and vividly to patients and their relatives, and in doing so he must be scrupulously accurate; for instance, it is unfair and wrong to tell a patient that an operation is a slight one when the risk is considerable. It is far better, if it is possible, to give the exact percentage mortality of the operation.

It is particularly necessary that a surgeon should observe great accuracy when delivering lectures to students or nurses. He should use clear and unmistakable language. In reading clinical lectures I have sometimes been very much surprised at the indefinite language used by some of the teachers in our large hospitals. For instance, in a lecture on the treatment of patients after abdominal operations the students were told that vomiting frequently occurs; that the best method of treatment is to give the patient some bicarbonate of soda and water, that he will vomit it up, and that this will effect a cure. There is no indication of the amount of bicarbonate of soda, or of the quantity or the temperature of the water. Moreover, patients do not always vomit it up and if they do this does not always effect a cure. It is bad enough to adopt a slovenly way of speaking of professional subjects in conversation, but when it is a question of training the younger generation it is a fault of the first magnitude. If definite statements can be made, they should be made in plain and unmistakable language. If indefinite statements have to be made, as they often have to be, this should be distinctly explained.

In performing an operation the surgeon must be rapid in his movements, yet never be hurried. Rapidity of movement is essential; hurry may be disastrous. The movements should be rapid, neat, purposeful, and controlled. I am certain that the time occupied in performing an operation is an important factor in determining the result of it. The longer the operation, the greater the shock; this accounts in no small measure for the lower mortality of a skilful surgeon.

Of all the attributes that go to the making of a skilful surgeon artistry is of prime importance, and it is perhaps the most impossible of attainment. Any surgeon can make an incision 5 inches long on the surface of the body; many can make it in the right place, but there are few who can do it artistically. To say that they all do it in the same way is absurd; it is no more true than would be the assertion that all men hit a golf ball in the same way. Art in surgery is difficult to explain, but it is a definite and visible attribute and it is born in a man. A man who does not possess it by nature will never attain it, though by practice he may improve his method of operating. He may become a craftsman, but he will never be an artist.

The possession of all these various attributes - general and special knowledge, good health, strength, the power of quick decision and immediate action, thoroughness, the ability to perform rapid and controlled movements without hurry, courage, artistic skill - may make a competent surgeon, yet such a man may fail to become a great surgeon. To my mind the possession of the surgical temperament is essential for the making of a truly great surgeon. The surgical temperament is inborn and it is rare - hence the woefully small number of great surgeons compared with the large numbers of competent men. The rarity of the surgical temperament is illustrated by the following incident. A doctor who had previously acted as House-Surgeon for me was staying at a hotel in a seaside resort. He got into conversation with another man who was staying there and found that he too was a doctor. In the course of their conversation they discussed the subject of surgeons. His acquaintance said to my friend, "How few surgeons there are who possess the surgical temperament!"

He had had an extensive experience of surgeons, yet he said he knew of only one man in the kingdom who possessed the true surgical temperament. My ex-House-Surgeon replied, "I quite agree with you, but I know another man who has it in a marked degree." The acquaintance then said, "Oh! What part of the country do you come from?" "Worcestershire," was the reply. "Then your man is Lionel Stretton, of Kidderminster, and he is mine too," said the other. It seems to me very remarkable, because I did not know the man, but apparently he had heard of me. I felt very highly complimented by the opinion of my former House-Surgeon, for he had been trained under some of the most eminent surgeons in the kingdom and yet he singled me out as the man possessing the surgical temperament. Of course I do not tell this story in any boastful spirit. The possession of the temperament is no credit to me; I did not acquire it, I was born with it. When I am operating I never feel the excited thrills that appear to affect many surgeons.

It is the surgical temperament that enables a man to adapt himself to any surroundings, to make good use of such assistants and instruments as are available, and never to be upset by any contretemps that may occur. The characteristics of this temperament are coolness, calmness, collectedness. If the anaesthetist, the principal assistant, or any other, collapses in a faint - this has happened several times when I have been operating - the surgeon should remain cool, serene, and collected, issue his orders quietly and carry on with the operation. If the condition of a patient becomes desperate during an operation it is even more important that the surgeon should remain calm, so that he may make every effort to resuscitate him. I often meet a man whose heart-beats and breathing stopped during an operation. By rapidly opening his abdomen and massaging his heart I was able to resuscitate him and then I completed the operation.

If death occurs during an operation and other patients are waiting to be operated upon these operations should be performed without delay. Some people consider this callous conduct. I consider it would be inhumane to postpone operations upon people who have been prepared for them. The man who makes an outward display of distress does no good to the relatives of the deceased, and he acts to the disadvantage of other patients. The man who controls himself is able to render effective service, though he often feels and suffers more acutely than the one who shows signs of distress. To possess the surgical temperament does not mean that a man is devoid of feeling, but it gives him power to keep his emotions under control and devote himself entirely to the work in hand. A man who wears his heart on his sleeve may give way to emotions that are gratifying to some of the relations at the time of a catastrophe, but he will go away and quickly forget all about it. A man with the surgical temperament will control his feelings while trying to comfort the relatives; he will go away to think over the case and try to profit by its lesson, perhaps to improve his technique and to think of methods to lessen the anguish of the distressed relatives. While he is lying awake at night considering these questions the emotional man will probably be peacefully slumbering.

The surgical temperament is particularly valuable when operations are performed upon prominent persons, especially in limited communities. A surgeon should be able to look upon all his patients as equally important. When King Edward had his operation for appendicitis several people remarked to me what a great responsibility and a great ordeal it must have been for the surgeon who operated upon him. My reply was, "Nothing of the kind, if he has got the surgical temperament." A surgeon who lives and works in a limited community, as I have done, knows that all eyes are upon him in the same way as they were upon the surgeon who operated upon the King; all his patients are kings, so to speak. He knows too that he must be prepared for criticism, and he hears the remarks that have been made about him. When I was collecting the money for the new operating theatre at the hospital I was told that it was said that I was asking for subscriptions for a new slaughterhouse! People are only too ready to say disagreeable things when patients die, but they often forget to say the pleasant things when they get well. The surgical temperament enables a man to withstand this kind of thing. If a surgeon has done his utmost and acted as he thinks right he should have no fear of what others may think or say. But perhaps the time when the surgical temperament is most needed and most valuable is when a man is operating upon his own relations and friends. The possession of it has enabled me to operate upon my nearest and dearest relations, which added very considerably to their comfort.

CHAPTER XXX

A BURNS DINNER

Scottish Society. Annual Burns Dinner. Toast of "The Immortal Memory." The eyes of Burns. Poetical genius. Burns night. Birth of Burns. His education. Mossgiel. Kilmarnock edition of poems. Edinburgh. Second edition of poems. Marriage. Ellisland. Appointment as Excise Officer. Dumfries. Songs. Death. Montgomery's appreciation. National poet. Humanity. Patriotism. English writings. His creed. His failings. Cause of death. Universal recognition.

Scotsmen are ubiquitous and consequently Scottish Societies flourish everywhere. This district is no exception and the local Scottish Society celebrates the anniversary of the birth of the national hero, Robert Burns, by holding a dinner on the 25th January every year. For many years I have attended that dinner as the guest of an old friend, a Scotsman and a member of the medical profession, who first came into this neighbourhood as House-Surgeon to the Hospital and later established a private practice a few miles away.

This year (1939) the Scottish Society honoured me with an invitation to the dinner as their guest and paid me the great and very unusual compliment of asking me to propose the toast of the evening, that of "The Immortal Memory." Why they should have invited an Englishman to do this I cannot understand. At first I felt rather chary of assuming the responsibility, but I decided that it would be ungracious of me to refuse, so I prepared and delivered the following address.

"I rise with some diffidence in this assembly, so largely composed of Scotsman, to propose the toast of The Immortal Memory of Robert Burns, one of the greatest men of the Scottish nation. But his fame is not merely national; it is universal, for his poems are known and treasured all the world over.

225

"If Burns were standing before us now we should immediately be impressed by one remarkable indication of a striking personality - his dark, flashing eyes, of which there are many records. Sir Walter Scott wrote: 'His eye alone, I think, indicated the poetical character and temperament. It was large and of a dark cast, which glowed when he spoke with feeling or interest. I never saw such another eye in a human head, though I have seen the most distinguished men of my time.'

"The majority of men are forgotten five years after their death; there are very few great men who are commonly spoken of one hundred years after their death. But your hero is commonly spoken of nearly 150 years after his death and will be commonly spoken of for all time; for he was possessed of a genius that enabled him to write poems that have been handed down, and will continue to be handed down, for the benefit of the human race. These poems stand out as a beacon light amid the flood of literature that the world has produced.

"On the 25th January every year, wherever there is a Scot - and where in the world is there not one? - Robert Burns will be remembered with gratitude and honour; for this is Burns night, and the anniversary of his birth 180 years ago. It is said that wherever there are two Scotsman - even in the remotest corners of the world - there is a Burns Society, and that it never fails to celebrate Burns night.

"The main facts of Burns' life are no doubt well known to all of you and there is no need to relate them in great detail.

"As you know, Robert Burns was born on the 25th January, 1759, in a cottage at Alloway, about two miles from the town of Ayr. His father was a working gardener and cottar, who built his cottage with his own hands, of the only materials at his command - mud, clay, stones, and straw. Today this clay-built cottage, rescued from unworthy hands and carefully restored, is one of the world's show-places, visited by pilgrims from all parts, coming to do homage to the gardener's immortal son.

"It is a common fallacy that Burns was an uneducated ploughman who by his own unaided genius produced marvellous poetry. It is true that he knew little Latin and no Greek, but he was taught English well, principally by John Murdoch, who was a born teacher. Burns is an example of the true Scottish spirit, which achieves education in spite of almost insuperable difficulties. He had only about four years' regular schooling, but he proved how much can be learned in a short time by an intelligent pupil when taught by a skilful ardent teacher who does not attempt too many subjects.

"When Burns was twenty-five he and his brother Gilbert took a farm of over 100 acres, known as Mossgiel. It did not produce much; the only thing that developed there seems to have been Burns' own poetical genius. It was there that he wrote the scathing satires against religious intolerance that first made him known as a poet. At about the same time he produced The Cottar's Saturday Night, a very different poem, in which he lovingly describes the household of his father and shows a keen sympathetic appreciation of the true religion to be found in the humble home of a Scottish peasant.

"After four unsuccessful years at Mossgiel Burns thought to make his way by going as manager to a sugar-cane plantation in the West Indies. To raise the money needed to pay for his passage his brother suggested that his poems should be printed. A small volume was therefore published (600 copies) in 1786 - the famous Kilmarnock edition, for which Burns received £20. It is interesting to note that within recent years a copy of this Kilmarnock edition was sold at Sotheby's, London, for £1,300. What a godsend that money would have been to the poet in his poverty!

"A contemporary of Burns, Robert Heron, who was living in Galloway when the Kilmarnock edition was published, states that 'old and young, high and low, learned and ignorant, were alike transported with the poems, and even ploughmen and maid-servants would gladly have bestowed the wages they earned, if they but might procure the works of Burns.' So eagerly was the book sought after that, where copies of it could not be obtained, many

227

of the poems were written out and sent round among admiring circles.

"When Burns was on the point of leaving for the West Indies he received an invitation to go to Edinburgh, which he accepted. During the winter of 1786 he became the lion of a season among the highest circles in Edinburgh, where he amazed everybody by his great conversational gifts, his manly bearing, and his mental power and independence of thought. A second edition of his poems was published in Edinburgh in 1787. For this he received nearly £600 and he at once sent £200 to his brother - a mark of his generosity. He spent the summer of the next year in travelling through Scotland, everywhere welcomed and honoured. He then returned to Edinburgh for the winter; but the learned and aristocratic circles that had previously entertained and feted him now received him coldly, and he left Edinburgh in the spring of 1788 an embittered and disappointed man.

"He then married Jean Amour, his faithful sweetheart, and took her to a new home, the farm of Ellisland in Dumfriesshire. Here again he was followed by misfortune. He was a good farmer and a hard worker, and those who worked under him testified to his sober habits; but the farm was too big for a family holding and too small for a full-scale farm, and it could not be made to pay.

"While Burns was at Ellisland he wrote Tam o' Shanter, which is recognised by himself and others as his masterpiece. It was founded on a legend of Galloway and was included in a book on the antiquities of Scotland published by Captain Grose. The poem was written in the winter of 1790 and was begun and ended in one day.

"To help to increase his income while still at the farm Burns undertook the work of an Excise Officer, but this had no good results. The pay was only £50 a year and his necessary absences from home led to neglect of the farm work.

"In 1791 Burns was appointed to the Dumfries division of the Excise, which yielded £70 a year. He and his family left the farm and moved to a small house in Dumfries; but the change from his beloved countryside did him no good physically, and he was more surrounded by temptations.

"He lived only five years longer, in poverty and ill health. Yet it was in this period that he produced the ripest fruit of his lyrical genius - a wealth of songs unrivalled in the literature of the world. He contributed more than two hundred songs to two collections of Scottish songs compiled respectively by Johnson and Thomson. These songs were priceless, yet Burns received no remuneration for them. No wonder he was poor!

"He died on the 21st July, 1796, aged 37½ years, in a poor house in a back street in the town of Dumfries. His funeral was a public one, attended by a great multitude; and a large sum was raised by subscription for his widow and four sons. A complete edition of Burns' works, including his correspondence, was published in 1800 and realised a sum of £1,400 for his widow and family.

"James Montgomery, a religious poet (1771 - 1854) whose name is now almost forgotten, left a very fine appreciation of Burns:-

> 'He passed through life's tempestuous night,
> A brilliant, trembling Northern Light,
> Through after years he shines from far,
> A fixed unsetting Polar Star.'

"Burns was his nation's poet. His poems contain inimitable descriptions of the manners, customs, and characteristics of his countrymen, all expressed in language understood by all, going straight to the heart of the people for whom he sang.

"The secret of Burns's world-wide influence lies in his humanity. His poetry shows the deepest sympathy with all the troubles, and the widest toleration for all the failings, of humanity. Burns is the absolutely natural man. He has been called Robert Everyman as Everyman would be if he could sing. He was a labourer, singing at his work. He was a lover - incurable and unrepentant - right up to the last. Does he not sing? –

> "The sweetest hours that e'er I spend,
> Are spent amang the lasses."

"Burns was also a thirsty man. He was surely a good customer of the inns of Ayr. Thirst has not disappeared. Thousands will wend their way on this festive night to numbers of well-lit inns - though the inns may be the Ritz, the Savoy, or the Swan of Stourport-on-Severn. They will eat their portion of the chieftain of the pudden race, accompanied by the wee drappie. '

"Burns is a natural patriot. To Everyman his own country means just what Scotland and Ayr and Bonnie Doon meant to Robert Burns. But he saw clearly that all local patriotism points inevitably to that wider patriotism, that independence of spirit, that proclaims the common humanity of common man:-

> 'Then let us pray that come it may -
> As come it will, for a' that -
> That sense and worth, o'er a' the earth,
> May bear the gree, and a' that;
> For a' that, and a' that, -
> It's comin' yet for a' that;
> That man to man, the world o'er,
> Shall brothers be for a' 'that!'

"Is it too much to hope that the day may dawn when all the nations of the world will agree with this, and act upon it?

"Burns wrote his best in the Scottish dialect, but he also wrote English in the most correct eighteenth-century manner. His finest English verses are those To Mary in Heaven, written on the third anniversary of the death of Mary Campbell, to whom he had been deeply attached.

"Burns' most wonderful legacy to the world is his songs. The greatest of all song-writers, he 'found a tune and words for every mood of man's heart.' Where else can be found the universal appeal of Auld Lang Syne? Hardly any English convivial social gathering that is held periodically is considered complete without the singing of this song.

"Burns' letters are valuable indications of his temperament and his beliefs. His creed was chiefly practical: 'Whatever mitigates the woes, or increases the happiness of others,' he writes, 'this is my criterion of goodness; and whatever injures society at large, or any individual in it, this is my measure of iniquity.' The same feeling he expressed in one of his earlier poems:

> 'But deep this truth impressed my mind,
> Through all his works abroad,
> The heart benevolent and kind
> The most resembles God.'

"On a cursory survey the known facts of Burns's life show that he had failings. No doubt he had, as we all have; but even so, it seems to me that he should not have been allowed to die in poverty and that his character and conduct should not have been condemned as they have been by many who ought to have known better.

"We may admit that Burns loved too well and too widely; and no sane person will waste time in denying that on occasions Burns drank deeply. But there is a world of difference between occasional out-bursts and continual tippling. In spite of the fact that 'not a man could be found in Dumfries who had ever seen Burns intoxicated,' in spite of the evidence, already referred to, of those who worked for him, and of the definite statement of his own wife, Jean Armour, that 'he never came home in an incapable state,' his first official biographer, Dr. James Currie, concluded that 'Burns died of drink and was a bad man.' It is significant that this conclusion was reached by a man who was such an ardent advocate of temperance as to be almost fanatical on the subject. How often have I known such extremists to be intolerant!

"Burns's writings prove that he was not a bad man, and evidence shows that he did not die of drink. He himself, as already mentioned, was most tolerant of human frailty, and our Great Master would assuredly have said to his detractors: 'Let him that is without sin among you cast the first stone!

"The well-known physician, Sir James Crichton-Browne, closely examined the facts and proved that there was no shadow of evidence that 'Burns died of drink.' The lethal effects of alcohol are unmistakable to a trained mind, and those effects were not observed in Burns. Sir James's considered opinion was that Burns died of heart disease, the result of rheumatism. Rheumatism attacked Burns in his early years; it damaged his heart, it embittered his life, and it cut short his career. This conclusive opinion of an eminent medical authority should be enough to end a scandalous and futile controversy.

"No man ever knew his own faults and failings better than Burns did. The verdict on this matter may surely be left where he himself left it:

> 'Who made the heart, 'tis He alone
> Decidedly can try us,
> He knows each chord – its various tone,
> Each spring – its various bias:
> Then at the balance, let's be mute,
> We never can adjust it;
> What's done we partly may compute,
> But know not what's resisted.'

"Burns' early death was one of the saddest in the whole annals of literature. But the last years of his poverty and neglect in Dumfries have been amply avenged in the full and universal recognition of his genius. Among all the brilliant sons of Scotland none is more honoured than Robert Burns, one of the mightiest poets that ever sprang from the people, and the most beloved.

"Let us then be upstanding and drink to the immortal memory of Robert Burns."

232

CHAPTER XXXI

MISCELLANEA

Sundry recollections and reflections. Worthy of Punch? An umbrella. Wild-goose calls. Abuse of hospitals. Family characteristics. Incompatibility in marriage. Unusual soap. Burst boilers. Generous impulses. Life Assurance. An air raid. Drunk or dying? Attendance on dogs. Importance of appearances.

In this chapter I propose to include a number of recollections and reflections that are recorded among my large collection of notes and do not exactly fit into the subjects of other chapters. Though more or less trivial, they may possibly be considered as not entirely lacking in interest.

Worthy of Punch?

One afternoon I was to attend the funeral of a man who had played an active part in the public life of the town. A friend who was to accompany me was having lunch with me beforehand and, rather naturally perhaps, funerals in general became the subject of the conversation at table. I said I did not like funerals; they were most melancholy and disagreeable functions. How much better it would be to be cremated! "I quite agree with you," said my friend; "funerals are horrid things. Remember that when I die you need not attend mine." Another friend who was present at once said, "Oh, but it would not be at all horrid for him to attend your funeral; it would give him the greatest pleasure." In a moment he realised what he had said and it gave us much amusement. We wondered if it was worthy of Punch.

An Umbrella.

I have lost a great number of umbrellas in my time, the reason being, I think, that I usually go out driving and have the habit of simply picking up my hat when I leave a house; hence on the rare occasions when I take an umbrella I am apt to forget and leave it behind. I once had as a birthday present a beautiful silk umbrella with a gold band on which my name and address were engraved. I soon lost it and did not see it again for five years. Then one day when I was coming out of a patient's house I saw my umbrella in the stand. I said to the lady of the house, "Why, there's my umbrella; I haven't seen it for years." "O yes, it has been most useful to us," she said unblushingly; "I hope you won't want to take it away." I felt very angry; I picked up the umbrella and found there was nothing of any use except the stick and the ribs, the silk being all in holes, but my name and address were still very clear. Some people have curious ideas of honour.

Wild-goose Calls.

I often see in the newspapers, in the account of an inquest perhaps, a complaint that the doctor did not come immediately he was sent for. If the public only knew the number of times a doctor is sent for urgently when he is not really required they would perhaps not be surprised at his apparent unreadiness to answer such calls. I have often been sent for most urgently when it was quite unnecessary. Here is an instance. I was performing an operation in the theatre at the hospital one afternoon when a lady who lived in a large house some few miles away telephoned that she wished to speak to me. I instructed the nurse to say that I was in the middle of an operation and I should be obliged if the lady would send me a message. Her message was that a youth had been caught in a threshing-machine and both his legs were torn off; he was bleeding seriously, and she would be glad if I would come to him immediately. I instructed the nurse to tell the lady that there were two doctors living within half a mile, that she should try to get one of them at once, and that I would be with her as soon as I could. I ordered my car, had instruments and dressings put ready in it, and as soon as I could complete my operation I took the House-Surgeon with me and told my chauffeur that we were going to a very serious case and he could drive at full speed. I have no doubt we exceeded the speed limit, though, incidentally, I have since come to agree with the statement that was made in the House of Commons when leave was sought to make an exception in our favour with regard to the speed limit, namely, that it could not be right to endanger many lives in order to try to save one. I think that

234

argument is unanswerable. When we arrived at the farmhouse where the accident had happened a car was standing at the door. It belonged to one of the doctors already referred to, and I found that he had been on the spot before the telephone message reached me. I sent to ask him if he would like me to see the patient with him. He invited me upstairs and told me with a laugh that there was only a slight wound about two inches long and he had put a couple of stitches in. The lady who had sent for me so urgently was a rich woman. If I had asked her for a fee she would have been most indignant, yet she had put me to the inconvenience and expense of this entirely unnecessary and useless journey.

Abuse of Hospitals.

Numbers of people who have money will not part with it if they can get something for nothing, and that is why hospitals are so much abused and the services of doctors are exploited. I maintain that if a patient possesses £1,000 he is not an object of charity, and he does not become an object of charity until he has spent his capital. Suppose such a patient has to have his leg off and dies as a result of the operation; it is obviously unfair that his relations should have that £1,000 and that the hospital that gave him shelter and nursing and the surgeon who attended him should go unrequited. If he recovers he should certainly be liable to pay for the medical attendance, and he could do so; it is only because it can be obtained for nothing that he does not pay. This is very well illustrated by the case of an old lady upon whom I operated some few years ago. I had to amputate her leg, which of course was done gratuitously, and she remained in the hospital several weeks. When she recovered she asked me about an artificial leg. I found out that she was living in a small cottage and receiving the old age pension, so I explained to her that artificial legs are very expensive and that probably she could manage without one. However, she was determined to have one, so I got the instrument maker to go and see her, having told him that he must explain to her about the cost, and that I could not be responsible for the payment. He told her that he could make her a serviceable leg for £8 to £10, but that if she wanted a better quality it would be £15 to £20; the best leg he could make would cost £35. She replied without a moment's hesitation that she would have the best. She had it and she paid for it. Had the hospital asked her for a guinea a week for the time she was in there and had the surgeon asked her for 10 guineas they would have been called robbers. Why? Because they give their services to those who cannot afford to pay, and therefore nobody can afford to pay if he does not wish to do so.

Here is another example of the same kind of thing. A man came to consult me and found that an operation was necessary. He went away to think the matter over, and a few days later I had a letter from him telling me that he had arranged to go into a hospital in London for the operation. He wrote that he would much rather have had me to operate upon him in my Nursing Home, but since he found he could have the operation performed for nothing at the hospital in London he preferred to keep the money to help to pay for a new Rolls-Royce he wanted. I have come across many similar instances. It is not really honest, but those who act in this way do not seem to understand that; at any rate let us hope they do not.

Family Characteristics.

There is no doubt that certain characteristics are evident in families. They are hereditary and include such traits as the conformation, the voice, the colour of the hair, the gait, and so on. Early marriage and longevity are also family characteristics and these are evident in my own family, as already indicated.

I have mentioned that very soon after I began my training at St. Bartholomew's Hospital I sent my cricket and football kit home. The men at the Hospital knew, however, that I had been an ardent football player, and one day they asked me to play for Charing Cross Hospital in a match. One of our reserve players was also a member of the Charing Cross team and as he was wanted to play for St. Bartholomew's they had to provide a deputy to play for Charing Cross in his stead. I told them I had not played for two years and I had no kit. However, they would take no refusal, so off I had to go to Twickenham. The Charing Cross men were very polite and asked me where I would like to play. I chose my old place, quarter-back, outside the scrimmage, and I got two tries for them in the first half. During the interval the man who was playing back for our side came up to me and said, "I was at school with you at ---- I knew this directly I saw you get that first try; nobody else could run as you do. Your name is Ernest, isn't it?" "No," I said, "it isn't, but my brother's name is Ernest and he went to school with you." That must have been a family gait.

Shortly after I went into partnership with my father I was in charge of the practice during his temporary absence. Among the patients I visited was a wealthy old lady who lived in a large house a few miles out of the town. A very stately butler admitted me to the house and, rather to my surprise, he ushered me into his mistress's bedroom saying, "Mr. Stretton, my lady," as he placed a chair for me at the bedside. It was a large four-poster bedstead with the curtains all drawn round it. After greeting the patient I began to make inquiries as to the state of her health, and a hand came out between the curtains so that I could feel the pulse. I asked to see the tongue and for this purpose I pulled the curtains aside. The patient gave a start and exclaimed, "I thought you were your father; your voice is exactly like his."

Incompatibility of Married People.

I have often been called upon to mediate between married people. There is generally a good reason for their incompatibility. Sometimes the husband is to blame, sometimes the wife, sometimes both are at fault; but I am convinced that once they have come to an open rupture it is much better for them to separate. I once negotiated a separation where the consideration paid to the wife was £600 a year, on condition that she kept away from her husband and did not molest him in any way. He pre-deceased her and when his will came to be examined it was found that he had left her £300 a year. If she had been my wife I think I might have felt inclined to shoot her, for she was a most exasperating woman. But for her husband to leave her only half what he had agreed to give her appears to me a most dishonourable act, and I cannot understand the attitude of mind that could allow it. There was no clause in the agreement as to what she was to have in case of his death. It is very difficult to provide for every eventuality, but I think that solicitors when drawing up such agreements should take care to safeguard their clients in every way.

Unusual Soap.

I was called out in the middle of one night by a doctor who had a confinement case that he was unable to deal with. When I arrived at the house I found only a dim lamplight. The doctor and the nurse were there and a basin of hot water had been put ready for me on the wash-hand-stand. I took off my coat and rolled up my sleeves to get a good wash. I picked up the soap from the soap-tray and proceeded to scrub my hands. I thought the soap felt rather hard and uneven and as no lather came I examined it more closely; I found that I had been trying to wash my hands with the patient's artificial teeth.

Burst Boilers.

There is often trouble owing to burst boilers and the difficulty of getting new ones. One would have thought that hot-water engineers would always have boilers in stock, but they rarely have. During the war it was almost impossible to get one. A boiler burst at the hospital and we were nearly a month without hot water there; they could not get a boiler of any kind. It so happened that two or three months before a boiler had burst at my house. Instead of waiting I put a man in a car and sent him over to a hot-water engineer and told him he was not to come back without a boiler of some kind or other, with the result that within forty-eight hours I had got my bath going again. I therefore told the Committee at the hospital that if they would leave it to me I was sure I could get a boiler, and I did. I persuaded one of the manufacturers to lend me his motor-van; I had to provide the petrol myself for it could not be got otherwise. I sent the same man as before on a journey of fifty miles and he brought the boiler back with him.

Generous Impulses.

A curious thing about human nature is that people are subject to generous impulses but do not always carry them out. I attended a certain doctor for many years and, as is the custom in the profession, I made no charge. His wife was so grateful to me for all I had done for him that when he died she asked me to choose amongst several articles what I would accept as a present from her. I made my selection and she said she would have it sent to my house. Knowing the frailty of human nature I said I would not trouble her to send it; I could easily take it with me in my car. But she would not allow that and said she wanted to have it cleaned up properly before I had it. It has never arrived.

Another patient, an old lady whom I had attended for several years, was very much attached to me. When she was dying she ordered the nurse out of the room and then said to me: "Now I wish to thank you for all your devotion and skill, and please kiss me," which I did. She then told me she was so anxious that I should have something to remind me of her that she had instructed her sons (both of whom were rich men) to give a special book to me after her death. Her estate was not a large one - perhaps between £5,000 and £10,000. Her sons divided it between them, but they never gave me that book. An old lady patient presented my father with a cow the day before she died, her companion being present when she made the gift My father and his coachman went to inspect the cow, and the coachman suggested that he should drive the animal home and my father should mount on the box of the Brougham and drive himself home. This he refused to do. The cow was not removed, the old lady died the next day, and her executors repudiated the gift.

Life Assurance.

I consider it is the duty of every man who marries to assure his life, and unless he can do this he ought not to marry. The whole object of the life assurance is to give the best possible cover for his widow in the event of his early death. The amount of the assurance must be decided in accordance with the position that he allows his wife to assume. If he and his wife are spending £500 a year I consider that it is nothing short of cruelty to leave her with a policy for £1,000, which will at the most bring her in £50 a year after his death. I once discussed this question with a patient of mine who was spending somewhere about £500 a year. I asked him if he was adequately assured and he told me that he was well covered. When he died, within the next two or three years, he left a widow and two young children with a policy of assurance for £500 and nothing else to support them.

I have always prided myself on the fact that I could put my head on the pillow when I went to bed at night with the full knowledge that if I died during that night my wife would have enough to bring up her family in that position in which we were living. To do this entails some sacrifice but it is well worth doing. I am referring to the man who has no capital, and particularly to the professional man whose capital is contained in his brain, which must die with him. Surely if a race-horse is worth insuring for £20,000 (and some of them have been insured for more than double that) a young professional man is potentially as valuable, even looked at from the commercial point of view.

An Air Raid.

When the air raids were going on during the Great War some German Zeppelins came within a mile of Kidderminster one night. I was due to give a lecture to the nurses at the hospital. I had been warned about the raid but I walked up to the hospital from my house, wondering whether a bomb would drop while I was on the way. When I arrived at the hospital the Matron, who was a most capable, self-possessed woman, met me in the hall and asked me what I had come for. When I said, "To deliver my lecture," she exclaimed, "Oh, but that's impossible! None of the nurses could listen to it; they are all too terrified. Haven't you heard that an air raid is going on?" I replied, "Yes, I have, and I should think that is just the reason why they should have their lecture; it will keep them quiet and give them something else to think about." I had them assembled in the lecture room and began my lecture with the aid of one candle, because there had been an order to put all the lights out. I had not been speaking more than a minute or two when there was a violent ringing of the bell; a police officer appeared and ordered that candle to be put out. I had it put out and continued my lecture to the nurses for an hour in the dark. When I had finished I told them they could now go quietly to their rooms and not have any fear. My surgical temperament was useful on that occasion.

Drunk or Dying?

Some years ago I was called in to see a prominent townsman who, it was alleged, had been found drunk and incapable. He was lying in the road after the licensed houses had closed at night and was picked up and taken home by two policemen. The doctor who was attending him called me in to see him the next day. He was suffering from arteriosclerosis. In due course he was summoned to appear before the Court and I gave evidence in his defence. My evidence was that he was suffering from arteriosclerosis, that it was not uncommon for people who were thus affected to have capillary haemorrhage in the brain, which would cause them to fall down suddenly, and that it was quite conceivable that he had had such an attack when he was found by the police. In cross-examination I admitted that I was unable to say whether he was drunk at the time, because I did not see him then. The only evidence of drunkenness was the opinion of the two policemen who found him. I told the Counsel who was defending him that I had instructed these men in First Aid, and I put into his hands a copy of my book containing the signs of drunkenness. I said to him, "I will guarantee that if you ask these policemen to give you the signs of drunkenness they will be unable to do so," and they were. They had no case and were obliged to dismiss the man. I further stated in my evidence that cases are recorded of men who had been arrested for drunkenness and found dead in their cells, from cerebral haemorrhage, the next morning.

This case created a good deal of interest in the town and some very uncomplimentary opinions were expressed about my evidence; it was even said that I had perjured myself. This did not trouble me; I had simply stated facts. It was an instance of the folly of the police at that period in not obtaining medical evidence of drunkenness at the time of arrest. I believe they always do this now.

An interesting sequel to this case occurred some few years later, when the man's brother-in-law got into trouble for being drunk while in charge of a horse. Of course he came to me to get him out of it. On questioning him I found that at the time of his arrest he had been seen by the Police Surgeon, who pronounced him drunk and incapable. I advised him to plead guilty and express his regret. What else could I do?

Attendance on Dogs.

In the course of my career I have attended some prize dogs that belonged to a patient of mine. She sometimes called me up in the middle of the night to see them. She always said they were exactly like human beings and that I treated them much better than the veterinary surgeon did. This reminds me of the story of a noted physician who was called up in the night by an artist to attend his favourite dog. The physician was indignant and not long afterwards he sent for the artist to his house and asked him to paint his front door.

Importance of Appearances.

An old lady came from the country one day to consult me. After examining her I found it was advisable for her to undergo an operation, to which she consented. The next day her two sisters came to inquire about her condition. They told me that the old lady was very much concerned because she was not going to be operated upon in London, where she had lived between forty and fifty years. "We discussed her coming to see you", said one of her sisters, "and it was decided that I should first come to Kidderminster and have a look at your house. I did so and went back and told my sister that I felt sure she would be quite safe in your hands." There is no doubt that if I had been living in a small house of insignificant appearance they would not have come to consult me.

CHAPTER XXXII

FINIS

Omissions. Views on surgery. Aim. Othello's injunction. Life work. Changes and developments. Hope for future.

This chapter brings my book to a close. Whether it will satisfy the expectations of the many friends who have urged me to write it I cannot say. I might have made it very much longer, written more about my family and private life, included many more of the large number of speeches I have made on different occasions, recorded some of the various so-called popular lectures I have given, entered into much more detail about my work, re-printed some of the many papers and reports of my cases that have been published in the medical press, given an account of some of the controversies I have engaged in. But all this I have deliberately refrained from doing.

I hold very pronounced views on certain subjects, most of all on surgery and questions relating to it, for after all that has been the main work of my life, and I have welcomed this opportunity of placing them on record. My aim has been to produce a book that may perhaps be fortunate enough to attract the attention of some few members of my own profession and yet not be entirely devoid of interest for the general public. I can honestly assert that it contains the truth, so far as I see it, and nothing but the truth, but I am not so presumptuous as to claim that it contains the whole truth. Indeed, that would be an impossibility for any book.

I have expressed indignation at certain things that appear to me to be wrong in general, some of them being discreditable to our great profession in particular; but I nurse no grievance and I bear no grudge against anyone. I have been mindful of Othello's injunction: though I may have extenuated nothing, I have not "set down aught in malice." I have had successes and I have made mistakes, but throughout my career I have tried to play the game. My work has always been as it still is - a never-failing source of interest and happiness to me, and the heavy burden of responsibility that every surgeon has to bear has been lightened by many proofs of confidence in me and appreciation of my work.

In the course of my long life I have seen and studied great changes and wonderful developments in the whole science and art of medicine. Great teachers and workers play their parts and pass away; but others are ready to step into the gap and hand down the torch of knowledge from one generation to another. The work of research goes on unceasingly and I cherish the hope that the future may hold in store still more marvellous changes and developments - discoveries that may bring to humanity benefits and blessings that are as yet to be seen only with the eyes of faith and in the light of imagination.

AFTERWORD

The front cover, from a photograph dated approximately 1898, shows Lionel with his wife, Lucy Emma and their three children: Rosa Marguerite, born 8th March 1885, Samuel Houghton, born 5th March 1886 and John Weston, born 21st June 1888.

Clearly the medical gene was well developed in the Stretton family as John Weston went on to follow his father as a surgeon in the same hospital, whilst John Weston's eldest son, my father, Lionel James, also trained at St Bartholomew's Hospital in London before going into general practice. With Lionel's grandfather and father this made five generations, all of whom trained at Bart's, surely a record!

Myself? I broke the long-standing family tradition, although I would argue that my career was spent in 'preventive medicine', having responsibilities for the production of safe drinking water to thousands of people throughout large parts of Wales for many years.

The introduction of tincture of iodine to surgery was a hugely significant event in the history of medicine and I believe Lionel has not yet received the recognition that should be due for this achievement. Not only did it revolutionise surgery but iodine became common-place in everyone's medicine cabinet and, in the Second World War, there was an ampoule of iodine in every soldier's field dressing. In the appreciation article, published in the national newspaper, the Sunday Dispatch, immediately after Lionel's death in 1943 and reproduced in Addenda 7.3, the journalist asks a 'senior medical friend', "Was not this a tremendous contribution to medicine? Ought not Mr Stretton to be almost as well known as Lister?". "Undoubtedly" he replied.

With three generations of Stretton surgeons at Kidderminster hospital, spanning the years 1856 to 1953, their influence has been substantial and, as noted in the Foreword, you can learn more of Lionel, his father and son in the book entitled "Dr Stretton, I presume" written by Kidderminster's local historian, Nigel Gilbert.

ADDENDA

ADDENDUM 1

INTRODUCTION OF TINCTURE OF IODINE

1-1   The sterilization of the skin of operation areas
      The British Medical Journal – August 14 1909

1-2   The sterilization of the skin of operation areas
      The British Journal of Nursing – August 21 1909

1-3   A further contribution on the sterilization of the skin of operation areas
      The British Medical Journal – June 4 1910

1-4   A further contribution on the sterilization of the skin of operation areas
      The British Medical Journal – May 22 1915

1-5   Letter clarifying credit for introduction
      The Lancet – September 3 1910

1-6   Letter clarifying credit for introduction
      The Lancet – January 14 1911

1-7   Letter from H Goodwyn claiming credit for introduction
      The British Medical Journal – November 18 1911

1-8   Letter replying to H Goodwyn
      The British Medical Journal – November 25 1911

1-9   Letter regarding introduction
      The British Medical Journal – August 18 1915

1-10 Letter: shaving the vulva
      The British Medical Journal – February 2 1925

Acknowledgements are made to
   The British Medical Journal and The Lancet
   for permissions to reproduce these documents.

Addendum 1-1

368   THE BRITISH MEDICAL JOURNAL]   STERILIZATION OF THE SKIN.   [AUG. 14, 1909.

A NOTE ON PROGNOSIS IN TETANUS.

By JOHN PATON, M.D.,

DISPENSARY SURGEON, AND SURGEON TO SEPTIC WARDS, VICTORIA INFIRMARY.

THE undernoted cases admitted to the septic wards present some points of interest. Both were under treatment or observation when symptoms of tetanus appeared. Antitetanus serum was used freely in each, and yet the course of the disease and the results of the treatment were quite different.

The following histories are founded on the notes made by Drs. Muir and Sinclair respectively:

CASE I.—J. K., aged 52, miner, was admitted on January 6th, 1909, with a large fungating mass on the outer aspect of the left thigh of two years' duration. He complained more, however, of pain in the stomach of a fortnight's duration. A large tender swelling was found in the hypogastric and left iliac regions. The patient looked ill and perspired freely. An enema was given with little result; the bowels had not moved for four days. Pulse 111, temperature 100.6°. The patient gives a history of having been in the Royal Infirmary two months earlier, when he was advised to have the leg amputated. I found marked tenderness and rigidity of the abdomen, and rigidity also of the muscles of the lower jaw and of the extremities. He was given a dose of croton oil and an injection of antitetanus serum. Films were prepared from the surface of the epitheliomatous mass, which showed the tetanus bacillus in large numbers. Under treatment by antitetanus serum and the daily application of hydrogen peroxide the rigidity gradually passed away, and by February 5th we were able to disarticulate the leg at the hip. The patient is now well.

CASE II.—J. K., aged 38, calendar finisher, was admitted on April 18th, 1909, from the dispensary, complaining of stiffness of the jaw and back of the neck of one day's duration. On Saturday, April 10th, he fell on the point of his thumb, which he dislocated at the interphalangeal joint; the skin was broken, and the head of the second phalanx protruded through the aperture. Evidently the parts had been for about an hour in this state before he came to hospital. At the dispensary the finger was steeped for half an hour in 1 in 40 carbolic solution. The dislocation was then reduced and a wet dressing applied. The finger had been dressed daily since. Suppuration started in the finger, which became red, swollen, tense, and painful. On April 17th the opening at the joint was enlarged downwards to allow the pus to escape. On admission the patient was complaining of pain in the upper left part of the abdomen and there was marked rigidity of the abdominal wall. The legs and arms were not rigid. The bowels had not moved for three days. Pulse 120, temperature 99°. Nasal feeding was tried, but was unsuccessful. An enema was also given without result; 30 grains of chloral were administered per rectum, with a nutrient enema of peptonized milk. On April 19th, in the morning, he had a spasm. Chloroform was given, and during the administration pulse and respiration ceased, but were ultimately re-established. Nutrient suppositories were given every two hours. At 9.15 a.m. next day he had another spasm. He became cyanosed, and respiration was difficult. The pulse became weak and could hardly be felt. There was not marked opisthotonos. Shortly after this the pulse could not be felt and the respirations stopped. The patient died at 9.30.

On comparing these cases it seems evident that the difference in the result was due to the difference in the site of the infection and the resulting difference in the facility for multiplication afforded to the bacillus. In Case II on post-mortem examination pus was found in the tendon sheath, extending to the elbow, a condition which could not be diagnosed clinically, and was not even anticipated by the pathologist, but found when looked for. In pus taken near the elbow the tetanus bacillus was discovered.

The conclusion to be drawn from these cases is that the synovial fluid of the tendon sheath is an excellent medium for the growth of the tetanus bacillus, and that steeping in 1 in 40 carbolic will not prevent the occurrence of tetanus if the tendon sheaths are exposed. When tetanus has occurred, also, the sheath of the tendon should be freely opened up, even although there is no apparent necessity to do this. From Case I also it is evident that hydrogen peroxide is capable of destroying the tetanus bacillus when it can be reached. Whether the antitetanus serum was of any value or not it is impossible to say.

I am indebted to Dr. Robert Taylor for permission to publish Case II, the patient being under his care.

The late Miss Annie Marples, of Broomfield, Sheffield, has bequeathed £2,000 each to the Sheffield Royal Hospital, the Sheffield Royal Infirmary, and the Hospital for Women at Sheffield.

THE STERILIZATION OF THE SKIN OF OPERATION AREAS.

By J. LIONEL STRETTON, L.R.C.P., M.R.C.S.,

SENIOR SURGEON, KIDDERMINSTER INFIRMARY AND CHILDREN'S HOSPITAL.

MOST surgeons will admit that occasional cases of suppuration occur in their practice for which they are unable to account. The most frequent are small stitch abscesses. They are generally attributed to the suture material, but I venture to think that such blame is often misplaced. Of all our preparations the one least under control is the sterilization of the skin. It is impossible to perform or even to supervise the process, and we are therefore dependent upon the assistant or nurse who undertakes the duty. The results we obtain prove that it is efficiently carried out in the majority of cases, but it is improbable that amongst a large number occasional defects will not occur.

The ideal method is one which can be inspected by the operator or one which will leave visible proof that it has been thoroughly carried out. If a substance could be discovered which would render the skin sterile when painted over it and would leave a visible stain there would be little chance of error.

Thinking of this I was much interested in an article describing the method of skin sterilization with iodine, as used by Dr. A. Grossich, of Fiume, in the EPITOME of the JOURNAL for November 21st, 1908. It was again brought before your readers by Major Porter on February 6th, 1909, and in the following week Mr. Goodwin informed us that it is used in the clinic of Professor von Eiselsberg in the Allgemeine Krankenhaus at Vienna. The method appeared to me exactly what I desired. I was, however, very sceptical as to its efficiency, and I could not bring myself to paint such a strong solution of iodine as recommended (10 per cent.) on the skin, especially as it was directed to repeat it twice. I have seen acute dermatitis follow a single painting—a condition I should not like to produce about an operation wound. It struck me that perhaps a weaker solution might be sufficient, and I accordingly decided to try the tincture of iodine B.P., which is about a quarter of the strength.

I commenced with minor cases, but I was soon so well satisfied that I extended it to others. During two months I have used it in upwards of 50 cases, the particulars of which are given in the table on page 369.

Where a "perfect" result is recorded, there was primary union without any suppuration, stitch abscess, or inflammation. In two cases there was some separation owing to deficient skin, which caused a granulating wound, but otherwise they healed immediately. Three of the goitre cases were discharged from hospital in a week.

The cases described as satisfactory were septic at the time of operation. The two cases of appendicitis were suppurative ones, requiring drainage. The colostomy wound was, of course, immediately subject to faecal contamination, and the same applies to the three colotomies, as they had to be opened immediately. All of them healed with a minimum of inflammatory trouble.

The ages of the patients varied from 2 months to 84 years. In none of them did the iodine application cause the slightest discomfort. The cases are fairly representative, and include some of the most anxious—knee-joint, fracture, hernia, etc.

If we disregard the 6 septic cases, there remain 51 consecutive successes and no failure.

The method I adopt is to paint a wide area of the surface to be operated upon with the iodine solution previous to the administration of the anaesthetic. It is painted on very freely, especially over hairy parts, and allowed to soak in. It is again painted immediately preceding the operation. After the stitches are inserted they are painted over for a margin of an inch all round.

The first and only dressing is usually made on the eighth day; the stitches are then removed, and the line of incision with a margin of 1 in. is painted with the iodine solution. If for any reason the wound requires to be inspected at an earlier date, it is painted as above described.

No previous preparation of any kind is undertaken—no bath, no scrubbing, and no shaving. The latter is an

Operations Performed with Iodine Skin Preparation.

Operation.	No.	Result.
Amputation, thigh	1	Perfect.
Amputation, breast	2	,,
Appendicitis	2	Satisfactory.
Appendicostomy	1	Perfect.
Colostomy	1	Satisfactory.
Colotomy	3	,,
Epithelioma of lip	1	Perfect.
Fracture, malunited	1	,,
Glands in neck	2	,,
Goitre	5	,,
Hernia, strangulated	1	,,
Hernia, radical cure	6	,,
Hydrocele, radical cure	2	,,
Incisions in fingers	2	,,
Injections of antitoxin	4	,,
Knee joint exploration	1	,,
Laparotomy exploration	1	,,
Laparotomy, mesenteric glands	1	,,
Laparotomy, ruptured tubal gestation	1	,,
Osteotomy, femur	1	,,
Paracentesis thoracis	1	,,
Plastic operations	2	,,
Trephining	2	,,
Tumours, subcutaneous	7	,,
Varicose veins	6	,,
	Total ... 57	

important point, because it saves the patient a good deal of after-discomfort. This is at variance with the method previously referred to, and combined with the weaker solution of iodine constitutes the difference.

The solution I use is made of 1 part of liq. iodi fort. B.P. and 3 parts of spirit. The spirit is made by mixing equal parts of spt. vini meth. and distilled water. It is practically the same strength as the tincture of the B.P., but is cheaper, owing to the use of methylated spirit. This is a consideration not to be neglected in a hospital where large quantities are used.

I have no means of verifying my results by bacteriological investigations, but practically they are so uniformly satisfactory that I feel justified in bringing them forward. My reasons for advocating the use of iodine solution are:

1. That it is an efficient method of skin sterilization.
2. The surgeon can be absolutely certain that it has been applied.
3. It is quickly and easily applied.
4. It saves the patient the suffering of a preparation which is at present very lengthy and very disagreeable.
5. It obviates the necessity of shaving, which is unpleasant at the time and causes considerable irritation afterwards.
6. It saves an enormous amount of labour upon the part of assistants and nurses, and consequently a lessened expenditure.
7. It saves the cost of preparatory materials and dressings.
8. It can be used in emergency cases where preparation by the usual method is impossible.

SIR FREDERICK TREVES has intimated that a scheme to bring the British Red Cross Organization into more intimate association with the Territorial Forces will shortly be issued. It is understood that the scheme will be carried out through the county associations and the county committees of the British Red Cross Society.

SEVENTY-SEVENTH ANNUAL MEETING
OF THE

British Medical Association.

Held at Belfast on July 23rd, 24th, 26th, 27th, 28th, 29th, and 30th.

PROCEEDINGS OF SECTIONS.

SECTION OF NAVY, ARMY, AND AMBULANCE.

Fleet Surgeon JOHN LLOYD THOMAS, R.N., President.

PRESIDENT'S INTRODUCTORY REMARKS.

IT is my proud privilege to extend, on behalf of the British Medical Association, a very hearty welcome to all who are present to-day at this Sectional meeting, and in particular to say how glad we are to hail, with friendly hand, those delegates who are amongst us from over-sea countries and who in that way join forces with us in what is the chief object of this—like all periodical meetings of the kind—research.

The British Medical Association, I need hardly say, is ever on the alert for and spares not any pains whenever and wherever the opportunity offers of improving the conditions which make for the advancement of medical and surgical science, and we of this Section, as a dutiful child of that Association, have our part to play, and I fervently hope that, during the next three days we shall have so conducted ourselves by inquiry and by free discussion of the excellent papers which are prepared for you on each day that the parent may not be disappointed in its offspring.

These papers show much devotion and keen perception on the part of the authors, and variety characterizes them.

For obvious reasons, individuality will be found in all such contributions, and sometimes the right meaning of the author may be a little clouded, and, of course, the opinions expressed are his own, and must not of necessity be accepted on that account; for these reasons, let us have free and friendly analysis, for wholesome criticism must make for betterment, even where a paper is originally good. The more the caloric the better the steel!

As the majority of those attending this Section are of the army or navy, and have in consequence been at one time or another closely associated with the medical officers of the various nations of the world, I take this opportunity of reminding the Section of the gigantic strides made, in this instance by our American cousins, in the realm of preventive medicine. It is only recent history how that Cuba, once the hotbed of yellow fever, has been lifted out of the Slough of Despond and been placed on a working footing with the other West Indian islands; this by the strenuous and most rigid observation of modern sanitary methods.

Much more recently, indeed at the present moment, the American Government is showing its comprehensive capabilities from the point of view of practical sanitation for stamping out once more that fell disease, yellow fever, on the arid and vast plains of Panama, where, in the days not far distant (when De Lesseps endeavoured to lay a course for its waterway), the white man found his grave, when the death toll generally was more appalling than we can afford to be reminded of with equanimity. Now, thanks to the glorious advancement of medical science, this veritable graveyard is again populated by white men (and women, too), who go about their business and make it possible for the engineers to face the problem of establishing a communication between the Western Ocean and the Far Eastern Seas.

Bacteriological research having taught us in recent years that *Stegomyia* mosquitos are the bearers of yellow fever, the destruction by the prevention of breeding of these pests, in addition to the most careful and studied protection

Medical Matters.

THE STERILISATION OF THE SKIN OF OPERATION AREAS.

Mr. J. Lionel Stretton, L.R.C.P., M.R.C.S., Senior Surgeon to the Kidderminster Infirmary and Children's Hospital, describes in the *British Medical Journal* the methods he adopts for the sterilisation of the skin of operation areas with iodine solution, which is a modified application of methods already described in that journal as practised by Dr. A. Grossich, of Fiume, Major Porter, and Professor von Eiselsberg in the Allgemeine Krankenhaus, Vienna. The method advocated by these authorities was to paint the skin with 10 per cent. solution of iodine, and this Mr. Stretton was unwilling to do owing to the tendency of iodine of this strength to produce acute dermatitis in some instances. He therefore decided to try the tincture of iodine B.P., which is about one-fourth of this strength.

Mr. Stretton writes, in part :—Most surgeons will admit that occasional cases of suppuration occur in their practice for which they are unable to account. The most frequent are small stitch abscesses. They are generally attributed to the suture material, but I venture to think that such blame is often misplaced. Of all our preparations the one least under control is the sterilisation of the skin. It is impossible to perform or even to supervise the process, and we are therefore dependent upon the assistant or nurse who undertakes the duty. The results we obtain prove that it is efficiently carried out in the majority of cases, but it is improbable that amongst a large number occasional defects will not occur.

The ideal method is one which can be inspected by the operator, or one which will leave visible proof that it has been thoroughly carried out. If a substance could be discovered which would render the skin sterile when painted over it, and leave a visible stain, there would be little chance of error.

The method I adopt is to paint a wide area of the surface to be operated upon with the iodine solution previous to the administration of the anaesthetic. It is painted on very freely, especially over hairy parts, and allowed to soak in. It is again painted immediately preceding the operation. After the stitches are inserted they are painted over for a margin of an inch all round.

The first and only dressing is usually made on the eighth day; the stitches are then removed, and the line of incision with a margin of one inch is painted with the iodine solution. If for any reason the wound requires to be inspected at an earlier date, it is painted as above described.

No previous preparation of any kind is undertaken—no bath, no scrubbing, and no shaving. The latter is an important point, because it saves the patient a good deal of after-discomfort. This is at variance with the method previously referred to, and combined with the weaker solution of iodine constitutes the difference.

The solution I use is made of 1 part liq. iodi fort. B.P. and 3 parts of spirit. The spirit is made by mixing equal parts of spt. vini meth. and distilled water. It is practically the same strength as the tincture of the B.P., but it is cheaper, owing to the use of methylated spirit. This is a consideration not to be neglected in a hospital where large quantities are used.

I have no means of verifying my results by bacteriological investigations, but practically they are so uniformly satisfactory that I feel justified in bringing them forward. My reasons for advocating the use of iodine solution are :—

1. That it is an efficient method of skin sterilisation.

2. The surgeon can be absolutely certain that it has been applied.

3. It is quickly and easily applied.

4. It saves the patient the suffering of a preparation which is at present very lengthy and very disagreeable.

5. It obviates the necessity of shaving, which is unpleasant at the time and causes considerable irritation afterwards.

6. It saves an enormous amount of labour upon the part of assistants and nurses, and consequently a lessened expenditure.

7. It saves the cost of preparatory materials and dressings.

8. It can be used in emergency cases where preparation by the usual method is impossible.

In 57 cases in which this method of preparation was adopted, in which the ages of the patients varied from 2 months to 84 years, the iodine application in no instance caused the slightest discomfort. In 51 cases the result was " perfect "—*i.e.*, there was primary union without any suppuration, stitch abscess, or inflammation; 6 cases, including 2 of appendicitis, 1 colostomy, and 3 colotomies, were septic at the time of operation. The results in all these cases were satisfactory, and they healed with a minimum amount of inflammatory trouble.

The method is one with which district nurses should be acquainted as the elaborate preparations used in hospital and private practice are often impracticable in the homes of the poor.

Addendum 1-3

1350 [The British Medical Journal] STERILIZATION OF SKIN IN OPERATION AREAS. [JUNE 4, 1910.

will do its work, and the other will, at any rate, do no harm.

The number of cases we give is, we think, sufficient to justify, at any rate, a provisional opinion on the subject, and we have no hesitation in using this reaction ourselves, and recommending it to the profession as a simple and harmless method of obtaining accurate information, which we have found to be of great value in many obscure cases.

A FURTHER CONTRIBUTION ON THE STERILIZATION OF THE SKIN OF OPERATION AREAS.*

By J. LIONEL STRETTON, M.R.C.S., L.R.C.P.,
SENIOR SURGEON, KIDDERMINSTER INFIRMARY AND CHILDREN'S HOSPITAL.

My first communication on the sterilization of the skin of operation areas[1] by iodine was based on an experience of 57 cases. A further experience of 291 cases has increased my belief in the method and enabled me to improve my technique.

In the accompanying table I have added my cases together, so that I can submit a complete list representing the operations I have performed during the last ten months which were suitable for such a preparation. The cases have

No. of Cases.	Operation.			Result.	Remarks.
5	Abscess			S.	2 healed per primam.
1	Amputation:	hip		S.	Was suppurating.
3	„	thigh		2 P., 1 S.	1 was gangrenous.
1	„	foot		P.	
1	„	hand		P.	
6	„	fingers		P.	
4	„	toes		P.	
14	„	breast		P.	
3	Anthrax			S.	Malignant pustules.
9	Appendix:	quiet		P.	
8	„	suppurating		S.	
3	Appendicostomy			P.	
1	Castration			P.	This healed per primam, in spite of secondary haemorrhage necessitating reopening the wound.
6	Circumcision			S.	
2	Colostomy			S.	
3	Cototomy			S.	
3	Empyema			S.	
2	Epithelioma, lip and face			1 S., 1 P.	
6	Fractures, wired			4 P., 1 S.	1 died (tetanus); 1 compound, some suppuration.
7	Glands in neck			6 P., 1 S.	1 was suppurating.
11	Goitre			P.	1 malignant, died in 48 hours.
1	Harelip			P.	
15	Hernia: radical cure			P.	4 femoral, treated with metal staples.
5	„	strangulated		4 P., 1 S.	1 was suppurating.
4	Hydrocele: radical cure			P.	
1	Ingrowing toenail			S.	Was suppurating.
6	Knee-joint operation			P.	
	Laminectomy				Died within 48 hours
12	Laparotomy: various			11 P.	1 after watery solution healed per primam; abscess followed.
1	„	extrauterine foetation		P.	
3	„	ovarian		P.	
	„	uterine fibroid			
6	„	ventrifixation of uterus		P.	
1	„	nephropexy		P.	

*Read before the Kidderminster Medical Society.

No. of Cases.	Operation.		Result.	Remarks.
1	Laparotomy : suture bladder		S.	Was suppurating; died.
7	„	gastro-enterostomy	P.	
1	„	perforated gastric ulcer	S.	Died within 24 hours.
1	„	gall stones	S.	
1	„	enterectomy	S.	Died within 48 hours.
1	„	intestinal anastomosis	S.	Died within 48 hours.
6	Mastoid operation		S.	
1	Nerve suture		S.	It had been suppurating; nerve held.
10	Naevus		P.	
3	Osteotomy		P.	
6	Paracentesis thoracis		P.	
3	Plastic operations		P.	
2	Ruptured perineum		S.	Healed per primam.
19	Small tumours; bursa, etc.		14 P.	One suppurated.
5	Sinus exploration		S.	All suppurating.
7	Tenotomy		P.	
1	Tendon suture		P.	
1	Tracheotomy		S.	
2	Trephining		P.	
36	Varicose veins		P.	
1	Varicocele		P.	
272				
	It has also been used in the following cases:			
23	Casualty wounds		S.	In most cases a perfect result; 1 gangrene, 1 tetanus.
27	Injection of antitoxin		P.	
25	Skin grafting		S.	
1	Vaccination		P.	Did not take!
348				

N.B.—In column three: P = perfect; S = satisfactory.

not been selected; they represent various classes of the community and ages varying from a few days to 84 years.

Of the 272 operations some were performed for conditions already septic, but from my experience of similar cases prepared by the former method I have no hesitation in saying that their after-progress was more satisfactory. They are marked as "satisfactory" in the table. Some have healed per primam and are marked "perfect."

I have had only three failures among the clean cases:

CASE I.—The first was an old man upon whom I performed an exploratory laparotomy. He was found to be suffering from malignant disease of the liver, and the abdominal wound was closed. When dressed on the eighth day, it was perfectly healed, and the stitches were removed. Five days later a collection of pus (about two ounces) was found beneath the cicatrix. This case was prepared with a watery solution of iodine, which I was then experimenting with. It is possible the failure was due to that, or there may have been no failure at all, and the abscess may have been due to infection from another source. This appears probable, because the skin wound healed perfectly, and there was no trace of redness about any of the sutures.

CASE II.—The second was the case of a small boy with a mole on his cheek, near the angle of the mouth, which I excised. It is difficult to apply a closed dressing in this situation, and it is still more difficult to keep it dry, in an adult; in a boy it is wellnigh impossible, and I feel satisfied that this was the cause of infection.

CASE III.—The third case is more difficult to account for. The patient was a man, aged 32, whose leg was fractured at football on March 28th by indirect violence. The left tibia was broken obliquely, and an x ray photograph showed about ¼ in. separation between the fragments.

On April 2nd I made an incision and fixed the ends of the bone with a screw and silver-wire suture. The operation was quite simple, and was performed in the usual way.

On the fourth day the temperature was raised, but when the wound was dressed it appeared to be all right. By the sixth day there was a decided red blush, which spread with alarming rapidity, and within twenty-four hours reached his groin. He was treated with Bier's congestion and injections of polyvalent serum (B. and W.). On the tenth day he developed signs of tetanus, which increased; he had constant convulsions, and died on the twelfth day. It is impossible to say how the infection occurred. If it was the fault of any of the preparations it is probable that the cases operated upon at the same time would have been affected. The ligatures used were catgut, prepared after the method of Sir William Macewen.

Suspicion was directed against catgut by Mr. W. G. Richardson in the BRITISH MEDICAL JOURNAL of April 17th, 1909. In the JOURNAL of May 29th, 1909, I reported a case of tetanus which occurred in a man eighteen days after an operation for varicose veins. The wounds had all healed per primam, and I was unable to account for the infection. I feel now, as I felt then, that there is no proof to connect them. The fact that this man was in a poor state, with a mouth full of decaying stumps, may have been, at any rate, a contributory cause.

Two or three other operations were performed the same morning under precisely similar conditions, including the excision from a man's neck of a huge carcinomatous mass, which necessitated the removal of the sterno-mastoid muscle and the deep jugular vein—a large dissection, lasting an hour and three-quarters. It healed up perfectly, and the stitches were removed on the eighth day, and he went home within a fortnight.

Besides septic and clean cases there are a considerable number which cannot be placed in either category. In such cases as appendicectomy and gastro-enterostomy, with the possibility of infecting the wound from the opened viscera, the skin preparation could not be blamed. Fortunately all these cases were successful and can be quoted in support of the method.

In cases such as circumcisions, where it is practically impossible to keep an aseptic dressing applied, healing occurs more quickly and there is less inflammation. Casualty wounds which have all been exposed to infection have in most instances healed perfectly. There were two failures—one a gunshot wound of the thigh which was followed by tetanus, and one a wound into the knee-joint followed by gangrene.

I tried the treatment in one vaccination, and I asked my friend Dr. O. C. P. Evans, the Public Vaccinator, to try it also. Our experience was very similar. It was too effective because it destroyed the lymph and there was no result, in spite of the fact that I allowed the iodine to dry on before performing the operation.

A former house-surgeon informs me that he finds the method useful for sterilizing his fingers in midwifery cases.

In this connexion arise the questions of staining, desquamation, and dermatitis. The staining does not persist, and I find that by the time most operations are completed all the colour has disappeared. If my hands become stained, as they often do, it is easily removed by washing them in a 1 per cent. solution of cyllin (3 per cent. carbolic solution is equally efficient), and towels are cleaned by soaking in a similar solution. There is no desquamation as a rule. I have seen it in one case, due, I think, to the solution being too strong, owing to exposure during a long operation and consequent evaporation. It should always be stored in a stoppered bottle, and only sufficient for use poured out. I prefer to use it direct from a wide-mouthed bottle. It can be applied with a sterilized swab or brush.

I am informed by several members of the profession that they are familiar with cases of acute dermatitis following the application of tincture of iodine, but personally I have not come across one. I have never heard any complaint of pain, and one house-surgeon who applies it freely to all casualty wounds informs me that there is no complaint.

My experience is that it is absolutely unnecessary to shave the skin, and this is an important advantage. Of all the preparations a lady has to undergo prior to an abdominal operation the shaving is the most repulsive, and during the period of convalescence the irritation of the growing hair causes great discomfort.

The only disadvantage I have discovered is lacrymation, to which some assistants are more susceptible than others. The tincture made with rectified spirit is far less irritating than that made from methylated spirit, and can be tolerated by most people. I still use the methylated spirit solution for the primary painting, which is performed immediately before the patient is anaesthetized. The second painting is done with the tincture when anaesthesia is complete, and the final when the operation is finished, with methylated. The tincture is of course suitable for all these purposes, but the increased cost is a factor which

has to be considered in hospital administration. To prepare a patient properly by my former method necessitated at least three days' residence in hospital prior to an operation. It occupied the house-surgeon or a nurse for periods varying from one to several hours, and besides all the chemical materials, at least two sets of aseptic dressings were required. The cost to the hospital on each case was considerable. On a large number a good round sum is saved in a year. What is still more important, the patients are saved the misery caused by these preparations. What is most important is that it is an efficient and reliable method, and the surgeon can always be certain that it has been thoroughly performed.

REFERENCE.
[1] BRITISH MEDICAL JOURNAL, 1909, ii, p. 368.

THE SCIENCE COMMITTEE
OF THE
British Medical Association.
REPORT CXXII.

A SOURCE OF FALLACY IN COUNTING RED CELLS.*

BY CECIL PRICE JONES, M.B.
(From the Pathological Department, Guy's Hospital, London.)

IT seems desirable to record some observations in connexion with red cell enumeration and the estimation of colour index, from which it is clear that the employment of Toisson's fluid for red cell counts is apt in some anæmic conditions to give very fallacious results.

I have prepared Toisson's fluid according to the following receipt: Distilled water, 160 c.cm.; glycerine, 30 c.cm.; sodium sulphate, 8 grams; sodium chloride, 1 gram. To the completely dissolved mixture I have added a few drops of a saturated aqueous solution of methyl violet to obtain the desired tint.

When counting the red cells of a rabbit which had been bled from the auricular vein on three successive days, I noted that the field contained, besides the usual red cell appearances, a number of very pale red cells, many of which were very difficult to see and readily escaped being counted, the result being an erroneously low red cell count and a correspondingly raised colour index. The number of these pale cells was increased with the interval of time after the mixing of the blood and Toisson's fluid in the counting chamber, and many cells became quite invisible with any ordinary methods of illumination.

The phenomenon was absent from normal rabbits' blood, but was observed in the blood of rabbits which had received phenylhydrazin subcutaneously. Table I gives some examples of this.

TABLE I.

Nature of Case.	Hb. per Cent.	Red Cells per c mm.		Toisson per Cent of Hayem.	Colour Index.	
		Toisson	Hayem		Toisson	Hayem
Rabbit X (normal) ...	89	5.40	5.61	98	0.63	0.61
Rabbit X after phenyl-hydrazin	32	1.30	1.60	75	1.34	1.0
Rabbit 27 (normal) ...	80	6.65	6.63	110	0.60	0.66
" " "	78	6.47	6.49	100	0.60	0.60
Rabbit 27 after phenyl-hydrazin	34	1.34	1.92	70	1.30	0.89
" " "	50	2.09	2.60	80	1.25	0.96
Rabbit 29 (normal) ...	84	7.05	7.05	100	0.6	0.6
" " "	86	7.27	7.07	103	0.59	0.60
Rabbit 29 after phenyl-hydrazin	28	1.06	1.49	71	1.3	0.96
" " "	38	1.53	2.11	72.5	1.26	0.90
" " "	48	1.93	2.43	83	1.23	1.0

* Towards the expenses of this research a grant was received from the Science Committee of the British Medical Association.

such attacks are, as a rule, materially lessened in frequency. When repeated quinsies have occurred, further attacks may be prevented by removing the source of the infection——namely, the tonsil. For lymphatic gland infections, where tuberculosis is suspected, tonsillectomy is indicated, and the course of the glandular enlargement determines whether more extended operative measures may be needed. In pyogenic infections of the glands the tonsil must be dealt with when the acute lymphadenitis has subsided or been operated on, if suppuration has supervened. Chronic glandular enlargement, of the mild or moderate degree, is so frequently met with in hypertrophied tonsils, that when the tonsil recovers its normal character the glands subside also. No tonsil should be removed when acutely inflamed. For more distant infections, when the tonsil is suspected of being the focus, removal is indicated when the general condition is satisfactory.

In all these cases total removal is the operation of choice; it presents no greater danger than incomplete removal, and can be readily accomplished by the guillotine alone, by a method first described by Mr. Whillis and myself in January, 1910. While these methods directed to the individual are of great importance, there is no doubt that prevention of tonsil infection should be our chief aim. This is to be obtained by the advances of hygiene—personal, in the home, and in the school. The maintenance of nasal respiration, the prevention of dental caries, and the proper supply of food, in sufficient quality and quantity, will greatly diminish the prevalence of this condition. The provision of a cleaner air supply and the prevention of infection by milk are measures needing attention. When that delicate balance between health and infection is upset, and the tonsil, a useful organ, becomes diseased and incapable of recovery, a timely removal of this focus may present more grave illness and disability. The question of infection of the tonsil and from the tonsil is not to be summed up in some form of operative procedure, but by attention to the numerous measures that have been indicated.

THE STERILIZATION OF THE SKIN WITH TINCTURE OF IODINE.

By J. LIONEL STRETTON.
SENIOR SURGEON, KIDDERMINSTER INFIRMARY AND CHILDREN'S HOSPITAL.

The method of sterilizing the skin with tincture of iodine which was originated by me, and which was first described in the British Medical Journal, August 14th, 1909, was received, as I expected, with a considerable amount of scepticism. In spite of this, it has rapidly gained favour and is now very widely adopted. The remarks which I read from time to time in the press make it evident that some of those who use it are not thorough in their methods; some adopt alterations and some deny that the method is efficacious. At such a juncture it may be well for me to state my further experience, to amplify my description, to emphasize the importance of some of its details, and to reply to some of the criticisms.

I have now used the method in upwards of 3,000 cases. It is unnecessary to publish a detailed list of these. It includes most of the operations a surgeon is called upon to perform. Among these cases I have never seen a stitch abscess, and I feel confident that the skin was in all cases sterile. Of course, I only refer to cases in which an aseptic result can be expected. You can hardly blame your skin if you find a Bacillus coli infection after the removal of a quiescent appendix! Even in cases which are septic previous to operation the skin incisions heal more surely and more rapidly. My extended experience has increased my confidence to such an extent that I never have any anxiety of skin infection. Of course I do not claim that it will secure asepsis in all cases. There are many other channels of infection besides the skin, some of which we may never be able to control. The one which always appears to me the most difficult is infection from within. Take, for instance, traumatic effusions of blood which have no direct communication with the atmosphere. How often they become infected! Or injuries into a joint without any breach of surface where infection supervenes. If by any chance a surgeon had aspirated such a joint before it became infected, few would believe that the germs entered by any other channel than the wound which he inflicted.

The solution I originally used was the tincture of iodine (B.P.). It is prepared by dissolving 2½ per cent. of iodine and 2½ per cent. of potassium iodide in rectified spirit. In an endeavour to save the funds of the hospital I tried a solution of the same strength in methylated spirit, but I soon found that it produced so much irritation and lacrymation that I was obliged to resume the original compound. I now use the tincture in the theatre and a similar solution made with methylated spirit in the wards. It was probably my effort to save the hospital funds which caused another surgeon to imagine that he had discovered the rectified spirit solution. He evidently did not read my paper carefully, or he would have learnt that my original work was done with tincture of iodine (B.P.), which is made with rectified spirit.

The method of application is similar to that which I originally described. A wide area of skin is painted half an hour before the patient is brought into the theatre. It is allowed to dry, and is then covered with a sterile towel. When the anaesthetic has been administered another painting is performed. It would be more correct to describe it as a rubbing, for I now use a small swab held in a pair of forceps, with which I rub the solution over the surface, taking special care over the hairy regions. If there is any occasion to increase my incision or to make a new one beyond the limits of the application, a further rubbing is easily performed. The little swab is dipped into the wide-mouthed bottle in which the tincture of iodine is stored, and if a further application is necessary a fresh swab is used. This is preferable to using a brush which is constantly dipped into the bottle. It has the further advantage that the stopper can be immediately put into the bottle, and so prevent evaporation or contamination. If a brush is left standing in the bottle this is impossible.

When the operation is completed the line of incision and about an inch margin is freely swabbed with the tincture. A sterile gauze dressing is usually applied, but in some cases, especially after hernia operations in children, no dressing is used. In septic cases I have packed in gauze soaked with the tincture. In all after dressings a free application is made. As a rule, the wounds are not uncovered for a week, but occasionally more frequent inspection is desirable or dressings are not applied. In such cases I swab with the tincture every day and have never seen any ill effect.

All the casualty wounds at our hospital are treated with it. Immediately they are seen a free application is made. After the necessary exploring, trimming, and stitching is complete a second application is made before the sterile dressing is applied. The improvement in results in these cases is most remarkable.

My patients are now admitted to the hospital the day previous to the operation. This saves them from the harass and distress of waiting and from the former elaborate and alarming preparations. The house-surgeons and the nurses are saved an enormous amount of work, and the hospital is saved the large expenditure which was formerly necessary for preliminary preparations. In twelve months this would amount to a very considerable sum.

Various modifications have been practised. Some have adopted a 2 per cent. solution, some an acetone mixture, and some a colourless solution, while others either wash the skin beforehand or paint on various solutions. I fail to see any justification for these alterations. If tincture of iodine is efficient, why alter it?

It was suggested that it was necessary to insist on a fresh solution for fear of decomposition, and then it was discovered that the formation of hydriodic acid which occurs if a solution of iodine in spirit is kept for any length of time could be prevented by the addition of 2½ per cent. of potassium iodide. These observers either failed to read my original paper, which states tinct. iodi B.P., or they forgot that the B.P. tincture contains 2½ per cent. of potassium iodide. If it is kept in a properly stoppered bottle, it will remain good for an indefinite time. If there is any evaporation, it becomes stronger and too irritant. Messrs. Oppenheimer have put it up in small wide-mouthed stoppered bottles properly sealed, which forms an ideal method of using it.

It is inaccurate to speak of the sterilization of the skin with tincture of iodine as the Continental method or to describe Grossich's solution as tincture of iodine, because his is a 10 per cent. solution of iodine in rectified spirit. It is almost identical in strength with our liquor iodi fort., which was formerly known as liniment of iodine. There is a very wide difference between that and the tincture. I would not use such a solution myself, and I do not believe any British surgeon would. I do not know if the skins of our countrymen are more tender than those of Continental inhabitants, but I am aware that a single painting with a strong solution (liq. iodi fort.) will produce acute dermatitis in many people. This is a condition no one would welcome in the region of a surgical wound, and for this reason, I expect, the method was not adopted in this country. It was not until after I had made my experiments with tincture of iodine and published my results that the method was adopted.

One surgeon wrote to me advocating a colourless solution because "it isn't so dirty." Surely stains are not dirty. As a matter of fact, I regard this staining as one of the important advantages of my method, because it defines the exact area of skin which has been sterilized. Previously we were at the mercy of a third person, and even if the duty was thoroughly performed—which I feel sure was mostly the case—we were unable to be certain where the boundaries were situated. If the surgeon's fingers become stained, the stain can easily be removed by washing them in a 3 per cent. solution of carbolic acid, or a ½ per cent. solution of cyllin.

I have never seen any dermatitis result from the use of tincture of iodine. There is sometimes a limited amount of desquamation. My experience is in entire disagreement with an observer who states that it is unsafe to use it in young children. I have many times applied it to babies, some only a day old, and I have never seen any irritation from it.

A question has been raised as to the pain caused by its application. Applied to the unbroken skin there is no pain at all, but when it is painted on a cut surface it produces a smarting or burning sensation, which rapidly passes away. It is so slight that some young children submit to it without complaint. I have made very careful observations on this point, and I have also tried the effects upon myself.

It has been suggested that it is dangerous to use it over the abdomen for fear of damaging the viscera if they escape and come in contact with it. I have no such fear; indeed, it is my custom to allow coils of intestine, etc., to rest on the skin which has been sterilized with tincture of iodine, and I have never seen any ill effect. I regard it as superior to sterile towels or gauze, because there is always a possibility that the process of their preparation may not have been perfect.

I understand that some surgeons still insist upon a preliminary scrubbing and washing. This is not only unnecessary but positively harmful, and the same applies to a wet compress applied before the operation. They both cause swelling of the epithelial cells and prevent the tincture of iodine penetrating to the deeper layers of the skin. It causes the germs to be shut up in snug little nests, and as the skin dries they are able to infect the wound. It does not signify how dirty people's skins appear. They come in from the works begrimed with dirt, sometimes positively black, but surely we need not fear a little carbon. Skins which look clean may be far more dangerous from a surgical point of view. If a bath is desired it should be given twenty-four hours before the operation. It is not necessary, and in some instances it is a source of additional discomfort and anxiety.

Some think this method of sterilizing the skin is of little use, and it is true that, so far, there is little bacteriological proof to support it; but the clinical evidence is so overwhelming that it cannot be ignored.

Carbolic acid may be stronger, but it would hardly do to paint it on the skin; to use it in the wounds must cause a considerable amount of destruction and sloughing. I do not think many men would care to use pure carbolic acid on an ordinary lacerated wound of the forearm and 1 in 20 carbolic outside. It would be difficult to prevent the acid getting out to the skin and burning it, and although 1 to 50

carbolic may be as strong as tincture of iodine, it lacks the penetrating virtue of the iodine, while it possesses the disadvantage of swelling the epithelial cells and shutting in the germs.

Most surgeons continue to shave their patients; this, too, is quite unnecessary. If it is done it should be done dry, or the swelling of the epithelial cells already referred to will be produced. In head cases there is so much hair, and it so hampers procedure, that it is best to dry-shave it; but in other situations it is quite sufficient to clip the hair away with scissors along the line of proposed incision. This is done when the patient is under the anaesthetic. The preparation as a whole is repulsive, especially to women, and shaving the privates is more objected to than all the rest put together. In addition to this, when the hair is growing again it causes irritation which is at times intense. To avoid shaving is another great advantage of my method—perhaps far more important than some surgeons realize.

I am pleased to see that the method is being used to a large extent on the battlefields, and I feel confident that it will be of great value. In emergencies of all kinds it is most useful. There is no looking up of basins or bowls which may or may not be septic, no crying out for sterile water which, if procurable, may contain germs, no mixing of carbolic acid, no nailbrush, no scrubbing. The simple application of tincture of iodine gives far more security. The surgeon's hands can be sterilized in the same way. I do not advocate it as a routine because the skin might not stand an unlimited use of it, but when it is necessary to use the hands so soon that there is not time to prepare them properly, it can be adopted with confidence.

That tincture of iodine is an efficient application for sterilizing the skin I am confident, and I wish that those who use it would adopt the measures I have indicated. This would add to the efficiency of their technique and save their patients a considerable amount of discomfort.

TYPHUS FEVER IN PALESTINE, 1913-14.

BY

C. H. CORBETT, M.B., Ch.B.Edin.

OWING to the havoc now wrought by typhus fever in Serbia it cannot fail to be of interest to report the salient points of an epidemic of this disease in Palestine, 1913-14.

Typhus is a rare affection in Palestine, and occurs in smaller or larger epidemics in certain localities about every ten years, and many physicians in the European or American hospitals in Palestine and Syria have never seen the disease. It is, indeed, highly probable that the epidemic of 1913-14 was the most widespread that has occurred in recent years.

In the spring of 1913, at the English Mission Hospital, Jerusalem, we were astonished at the virulence of the affection which was revealed to us by an infected family admitted to our wards.

This group of patients demonstrated the comparative mildness of the disease in childhood and early youth, whilst the severer type was witnessed in the mother. From these cases a nurse and a middle-aged ward woman became infected; the former recovered after a veritable fight for life, while the latter died—our only death in a series of not fewer than 20 cases.

Subsequently children and adults, individuals from various large families in congested and uncongested districts, received treatment; in all cases of adult infection a critical and anxious period was passed.

After we had attended to about 15 cases there was a lull in the storm, till Hebron was swept with the disease, and the exodus from Abraham's city reminded one of Lot's flight from Sodom.

Again there was a decrease in the number of cases while the coast towns received their spell of the pest, till, in the spring of 1914, I saw a Nubian boy in his house suffering from a continuous fever which I could only then diagnose as typhoid (his skin was too black to see a rash). He was admitted to our hospital on the ninth day of the illness, and was put on sodium sulpho-carbolates, grs. xx, every four hours. On the twelfth or thirteenth day he had the crisis, and I fondly imagined that a typhoid fever had been aborted. A few days later, however, his nurse

C

"SUBJECTS OF SURGICAL INTEREST."

To the Editor of THE LANCET.

SIR,—My attention has been called to a letter in your issue of August 20th on the above subject by Dr. Wm. Bennett of Manchester. In the course of his remarks he states that "general practitioners will thank Mr. Waterhouse for simplifying the disinfecting of operation surfaces." So far as I am aware, I was the first surgeon to advocate the use of tincture of iodine for this purpose. If Dr. Bennett will refer to the *British Medical Journal* of August 4th, 1909, he will find my original paper, which was published several months before Mr. Waterhouse's.

I am, Sir, yours faithfully,

J. LIONEL STRETTON,

Senior Surgeon to the Kidderminster Infirmary
and Children's Hospital.

Kidderminster, August 29th, 1910.

Addendum 1-5

The Lancet – September 3 1910

THE USE OF IODINE AS A DISINFECTANT OF THE SKIN BEFORE OPERATIONS.

To the Editor of THE LANCET.

SIR,—Will you permit me to inform Mr. Willmott Evans that he is in error in stating "the first advocate of its use in this country was Mr. H. F. Waterhouse." My original paper was published in the *British Medical Journal* on August 14th, 1909, several months before Mr. H. F. Waterhouse's communication. I there stated that Dr. A. Grossich of Fiume had used liquor iodi, 10 per cent. solution. So far as I am aware, I was the first surgeon to use tincture of iodine, 2½ per cent. solution. May I also point out that, as I have insisted, shaving is unnecessary and the colour of the iodine is an advantage because it shows the limits of its application.—I am, Sir, yours faithfully,

J. LIONEL STRETTON,

Senior Surgeon, Kidderminster Infirmary and
Children's Hospital.

Jan. 9th, 1911.

Addendum 1-6

The Lancet – January 14 1911

256

STERILIZATION OF THE SKIN BY IODINE.

SIR,—I note in the BRITISH MEDICAL JOURNAL of November 11th a letter from Dr. L. Stretton, in which he states he was the first surgeon to use tincture of iodine in the sterilization of the skin in surgical operations ; and I should like to point out that I wrote a short note in the BRITISH MEDICAL JOURNAL shortly before his paper appeared, referring to the use of this drug in Vienna in the hands of Professor von Eiselsberg in his clinic at the Allgemeine Krankenhaus, giving details of his results and stating the strength he used ; also I would refer you to Dr. Stretton's paper of the date quoted in which he mentions my paper. It is therefore obvious that he was not the first surgeon to use this method, as I had been using it for two years, and I think I am right in stating that it was entirely as a result of my paper that the method was adopted at the Middlesex Hospital under Sir A. Pearce Gould and other surgeons on the staff. Grossich's paper was the first published in this country, and his solution was 10 per cent. This is the strength used in Vienna, and, if my memory serves me, Dr. Stretton stated that he thought this solution too strong. I have always used this strength and have never found it produce any skin irritation, and skin abscess and stitch infection has been entirely absent. Apologizing for the length of my letter—I am, etc.,

H. GOODWYN, F.R.C.S.Edin.

Bovey Tracey, Devon, Nov. 12th.

Addendum 1-7

The British Medical Journal – November 18 1911

STERILIZATION OF THE SKIN BY IODINE.

SIR,—Mr. Goodwyn is evidently under a misapprehension as to the composition of tincture of iodine. If he will refer to the *British Pharmacopœia* he will find that it consists of 2½ per cent. iodine and 2½ per cent. potassium iodide dissolved in rectified spirit. When he describes the 10 per cent. solution which he uses as tincture of iodine, it "is obvious"—I use his own expression—that his description is inaccurate.

I have never claimed to be the originator of the strong solution, and I have acknowledged this in all my communications on the subject. I do claim to have originated the method of tincture of iodine, and this is the method which is now so generally used.—I am, etc.,

J. LIONEL STRETTON,

Senior Surgeon, Kidderminster Infirmary
and Children's Hospital.

Kidderminster, Nov. 18th.

Addendum 1-8

The British Medical Journal – November 25 1911

THE STERILIZATION OF THE SKIN WITH TINCTURE OF IODINE.

SIR,—If Surgeon-Major Porter will read my original paper, which appeared in the BRITISH MEDICAL JOURNAL of August 14th, 1909, he will find that I referred to the work of Professor Grossich. I also referred to his paper which was published in the JOURNAL of February 6th, 1909, and to a contribution by Mr. Goodwin the following week.

They had all used a 10 per cent. solution of iodine, which is known in this country as liq. iodi fort. or lin. iodi. Prior to my communication no one had ever suggested using tinct. iodi, *B.P.*

If Surgeon-Major Porter "quickly discovered that the 10 per cent. solution was not necessary and was sometimes injurious," he did not impart this knowledge to us, nor did he suggest an alternative method. I have never claimed to be the originator of the liq. iodi fort. method. I was the first to use and to advocate the tinct. iodi, *B.P.*, and this is the solution which is now universally used.— I am, etc.,

J. LIONEL STRETTON,
Senior Surgeon, Kidderminster Infirmary and Children's Hospital.

Kidderminster,
Aug. 9th.

Addendum 1-9

The British Medical Journal – August 18 1915

SHAVING THE VULVA.

SIR,—With reference to the letter of Dr. Henry Corby (January 31st, p. 235), in which he condemns the fashion of shaving the vulva during labour—I presume he means before labour commences—I agree with him that this process is unnecessary and that it is repulsive to most women.

I pointed this out in a paper entitled " The sterilization of the skin of operation areas," published in the BRITISH MEDICAL JOURNAL of August 14th, 1909. This paper describes the method, originated by me, of sterilizing the skin with tincture of iodine. In a further contribution on the same subject, published in the BRITISH MEDICAL JOURNAL of June 4th, 1910, I emphasized the point that the repulsive process of shaving is unnecessary. Since adopting the method of sterilization with tincture of iodine I do not allow the pudenda to be shaved prior to operation on the abdomen. All that is necessary is that the tincture of iodine should be thoroughly rubbed in. I have always found this effective.

A normal confinement is quite disagreeable enough without adding unnecessary discomfort. Such a process as shaving the vulva encourages the present-day tendency to evade motherhood; whereas we should do all in our power to encourage motherhood.—I am, etc.,

Kidderminster, Feb. 2nd.   J. LIONEL STRETTON.

Addendum 1-10

The British Medical Journal – February 7 1925

ADDENDUM 2

INVENTIONS

Acknowledgements are made to
   The British Medical Journal and The Lancet
   for permissions to reproduce these documents.

ENTROPIUM FORCEPS.

AT my suggestion Messrs. Arnold and Sons have constructed a pair of entropium forceps as figured in the accompanying illustration. It will be noticed that they are larger than the old-fashioned instrument and that they are fixed by a rack instead of a screw. This facilitates their application and enables an assistant to hold them in position more easily. The fenestrated blade is made to fit into a groove round the flattened blade and the

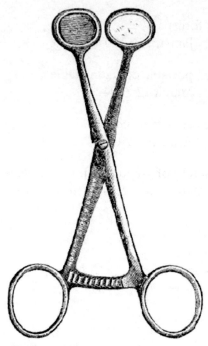

latter is made slightly convex so that it will force the tissues above the level of the fenestrated edge and save the scalpel coming in contact with it. In order that cleaning may be more thoroughly performed they are made with a detachable joint and the groove for the reception of the fenestrated blade is concave instead of angular. Anyone who has used the old-fashioned instrument must have experienced some of the difficulties I have indicated and as the removal of a tarsal cyst is an operation which many members of the profession undertake I hope that this modification may be of use.

I am indebted to Messrs. Arnold for the careful manner in which they have carried out my idea.

J. LIONEL STRETTON,
Senior Surgeon, Kidderminster Infirmary and Children's Hospital.

Addendum 2-1: The Lancet – January 30 1904

AN IMPROVED PORTABLE OPERATION TABLE.

THIS table is so constructed that it can readily be adjusted to the usual positions required. It is thoroughly substantial and rigid in each position and capable of supporting a weight of 20 stones; it can be folded into a comparatively small compass for carrying in a canvas case or satchel; it always folds up accurately and there is no likelihood of its being strained or bulged. When it is in its case it is not too heavy to move about with one hand. Its mechanism is so simple that it can be placed in the desired position or folded and put away in less than two minutes. It can be made in wood, polished or enameled, or in metal, nickeled or enameled, and is comparatively inexpensive. As shown in Fig. 1, it consists of a horizontal

FIG. 1.

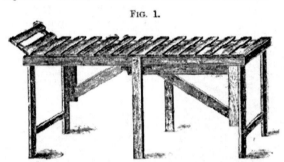

frame hinged in the centre; the legs and struts are also hinged and the cross laths of the table are so constructed that the whole falls accurately together. The Trendelenburg position, as shown in Fig. 2, is secured by lifting the table in

FIG. 2.

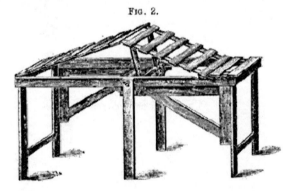

the centre and is maintained by a strut secured with thumb-screws. By a rack arrangement the portion corresponding to the upper position of the body can be raised to any position from the horizontal to the erect. If desired, a pair of crutches for the lithotomy position can be affixed to the lower end.

Messrs. Arnold and Sons of West Smithfield, London, E.C., have made the table at my suggestion and after 12 months' use I find it in every way satisfactory.

J. LIONEL STRETTON,
Senior Surgeon, Kidderminster Infirmary and
Children's Hospital.

Kidderminster.

Addendum 2-2: The Lancet – March 12 1904

New Inventions.

AN IMPROVED ADJUSTABLE COMMODE.

THIS commode admits of a variety of adjustments, in one of which it presents an entirely horizontal surface, as shown in Fig. 2. It will, therefore, sometimes be serviceable in cases where the bed-pan cannot be used. Its height can be adjusted to that of the bedstead. The seat is of a good size and shape, like an ordinary water-closet seat, instead of a small round hole as usually found in commodes, and it is so constructed that it can be slightly raised at the foot end and so prevent a patient from slipping down. The lid which forms the section for the support of the upper portion of the body can be placed horizontally or it can be raised to various heights so that a patient may sit upright or partially so. When raised it is retained in position by strong pieces of cable which form side supports so that it resembles an arm chair, as shown in Fig. 1. If a patient is too helpless to be supported in this way the lid can be folded back and an attendant can stand behind to give the necessary assistance. The section which forms the support for the lower extremities may either be maintained in the horizontal position, as shown in the illustration, or it may be folded down in order to allow the feet to be placed on a hassock. If desired it can be provided with a sliding foot-piece for this purpose. In cases where it is desirable to keep one leg only horizontal the section can be divided longitudinally so that one foot only is lowered. When not in use, the lower section hangs down in front and the upper section is folded over the seat, forming a useful bedside table.

FIG. 1.

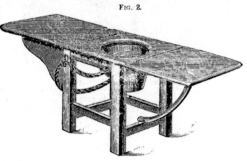

FIG. 2.

Messrs. Arnold and Sons of West Smithfield, London, E.C., are the makers of the commode.

J. LIONEL STRETTON,
Senior Surgeon, Kidderminster Infirmary and Children's Hospital.
Kidderminster.

Addendum 2-3

The Lancet – April 16 1904

264

that the mental condition was due to shock; and this view appears to have been correct. I saw him three months after he left the hospital, and he appeared then quite well.

THE MANUFACTURE OF ASEPTIC HOSPITAL FURNITURE.

By J. LIONEL STRETTON,

SENIOR SURGEON TO THE KIDDERMINSTER INFIRMARY AND CHILDREN'S HOSPITAL.

ALTHOUGH hospital furniture has been improved during the last twenty years, it is still far from perfect from an aseptic point of view. A considerable proportion of it has been made in Germany, and now that this source of supply

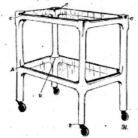

Fig. 1.—An operating-room table.

The angles A, A are all rounded and scalloped out. The socket carrying the castor is continuous with the table leg, so that no joint is visible, B. The rabbet holding the upper glass shelf C is scalloped out, though this is not seen in the photograph. The rounded and scalloped inside of the angles is seen at D.

is cut off, there is some difficulty in meeting the present increased demand.

At such a juncture I feel that it may be an advantage if I describe some of the articles which I have invented.

On examining some specimens of hospital furniture it will be seen that the manufacturers have left angles and depressions which act as receptacles for dirt and germs. It is difficult, and in some instances impossible, to clean them. I have endeavoured to guide some of the makers from their erroneous ways into the right direction. Hitherto my efforts have been without result; even when I have submitted models these have sometimes been incorrectly copied.

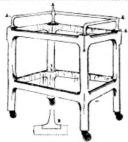

Fig. 2.—A ward wagon.

This is somewhat similar to the table, Fig. 1, but is of larger size and is provided with a metal rail, which has rounded angles at A, A. The feet are so constructed that they fit into the wagon, leaving a scooped-out edge, as shown in Fig. B.

Manufacturers appear to have adopted a stereotyped method of employing cornices, panels and ornamentation, and to be unable to avoid such adornment. Furthermore, they are not surgeons; they do not fully understand what we require, and they are consequently incapable of attending to the necessary details. It is equally true that surgeons are not furniture makers. If a perfect article is to be produced, combined effort is essential.

I have been fortunate in finding a local cabinet-maker able and willing to work with me and carry out my views. The drawings illustrate furniture he has recently con-

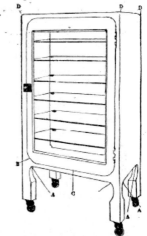

Fig. 3.—An instrument cabinet.

There is an entire absence of ornamentation. The angles are all rounded at A, A, A, and the same applies to all the inside angles. The bottom, C, is made to open flush, without any ledge to catch the dust and dirt, and the corners are all rounded as at D. The catch and striking plates are let in flush, and there is a spring stop in the striking plate to prevent a hole, which would contain dirt. The door is rounded at the corners so avoid angles, as at D, and it is bevelled down to the glass inside and outside. The edge is rounded, and fits into a scalloped rabbet. The glass shelves are supported by rounded metal plugs, which can easily be removed and reinserted.

structed under my supervision. These show my methods of construction, which it is difficult to explain clearly in an article.

Briefly, my object is to avoid any depression or angle—to make the furniture in such a way that the most

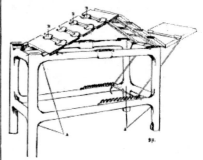

Fig. 4.—An operating-table.

The angles A, A, A are all rounded and scalloped. Where the cross pieces join, B, B, B, it is also scalloped. There are wheels on the feet of the table at the head, so that it is easy to move it about if the foot end is raised. The rack allows the head to be raised or lowered.

perfunctory dusting cannot fail to clean every portion of it.

To attain this end it is necessary to apply the above principles to the parts hidden at the back and underneath, as well as to those which are in full view. So far as I can judge, it is possible to obtain perfection in this respect—that is, to construct a piece of furniture without any receptacle for dirt.

All this furniture is constructed of wood and is enamelled white.

Some surgeons maintain that all hospital furniture must be constructed of iron. I understand that the argument in favour of this is that iron is non-absorbent. Do the advocates of metal realize that it is covered with a coat of enamel, and that it consequently becomes a question of this material? The enamel burnt on to metal is, perhaps, harder than the enamel on wood, but it possesses the great disadvantage of chipping. These chipped places provide spaces which form as commodious dwelling-places for germs as the caves in the rocks did for our ancestors. I have never seen a piece of enamelled metal furniture which has not chipped in a few weeks. and most of it *is* bespeckled before a year has passed. Enamel on wooden furniture never chips. There may be some separation of joints or a crack in the wood, but these can easily be filled with hard stopping. The furniture can be rubbed down and re-enamelled at intervals, after which treatment it comes out like new.

Wooden furniture is far lighter for moving about; it is strong enough for its purpose, and the cost is less than half that of the metal. I prefer wood. Those who retain an affection for metal could, no doubt, obtain furniture made after my designs.

The cabinet-maker who has assisted me is unable to manufacture any large quantity. Messrs. Salt, of Birmingham, assure me that they are in a position to do so.

Addendum 2-4
British Medical Journal – 30 October 1915

266

ADDENDUM 3

MEDICAL

Acknowledgements are made to
*   The British Medical Journal and The Lancet*
*   for permissions to reproduce these documents.*

ASEPTIC SURGERY.

Sir,—I have been much interested in reading the remarks of my friend, Mr. C. B. Lockwood, on Aseptic and Septic Surgical Cases with Special Reference to the Disinfection of Materials and the Skin, but I venture to suggest that the inconstancy of his results is to be partially explained by the fact that his tests are imperfect.

It is possible that a piece of material or sponge, "a scrap" of which has been proved to be aseptic, may still contain a multitude of germs, the more so if it be a towel with a hemmed border and the scrap have been removed from another place, but in case of the hands the possibility is transformed into a probability. "A scrap" of skin is hardly a fair specimen of so complex a member.

It seems to me that the positive evidence is of some value, because it points to the probability of its source being septic, but the negative evidence does not in all cases point to the probability of its being aseptic.

To render sterile the skin of the surgeon, of the assistants, and of the patient, together with the towel, sponges, and instruments, etc., is an ideal we should all aim at, and if Mr. Lockwood can devise an easy method of proving them to be in such a condition he would indeed elevate the position of surgery.—I am, etc.,

Kidderminster, July 13th.   J. Lionel Stretton.

Addendum 3-1

The British Medical Journal – July 18 1896

the thorax. Certainly, so far as they go, these figures do not support the idea that tuberculous meningitis is mainly due to the reception of tuberculous infection into the alimentary tract—unless, indeed, as is possible, the bacilli obtained access through the alimentary canal but without necessarily giving rise to any local lesion either there or in the mesenteric glands.

I am, Sirs, yours faithfully,

Cavendish-place, W., Dec. 6th, 1898.   J. WALTER CARR.

THE ANTI-TUBERCLE CRUSADE.

To the Editors of THE LANCET.

SIRS,—In a book written by Gideon Harvey, M.D., about 1660, consumption is described as an endemic and epidemic disease and the following passage gives some idea of the then prevalent belief in its infective nature: " And considering with all its malignity and contagious nature, it may be numbered among the worst Epidemicks or popular diseases, since next to the Plague, Pox, and Leprosie, it yields to none in point of contagion; for it's no rare observation here in England, to see a fresh coloured lusty young man yoake to a consumptive female, and him soon after attending her to the grave. Moreover nothing we find taints sound lungs sooner, than inspiring or drawing in the breath of putrid ulcered consumptive lungs; many having fallen into consumptions, only by smelling the breath or spittle of Consumptives, others by drinking after them; and what is more, by wearing the Cloaths of Consumptives, though two years after they were left off."

With the exception of the last sentence this opinion so nearly accords with the views of to-day that it is difficult to understand why it remained in abeyance for so many years. Of course it was not founded upon a scientific basis and, I suppose, as we became more exact we were unable to accept the clinical facts unless supported by experimental proof. Thanks to the discovery of Koch we are now emerging from the path of error into which we had temporarily strayed and in doing so I think we must admit that we should have been wiser, or at any rate conferred more benefit on mankind, if we had accepted the teachings of our predecessors who, if they had not the advantage of so much scientific knowledge to assist them, evidently possessed considerable clinical acumen and were able to make accurate deductions therefrom. There are, of course, errors in Gideon Harvey's book, but who can say that some of the statements are not in advance of even our boasted knowledge of to-day? As an instance we may take the reference to cancer as infective. Although we are still disinclined to accept it the disease affords us indications which support the view that it is to some extent communicable. The great factor which upsets all our calculations is the individual peculiarity which favours the development of a disease, and it is because we are unable to solve this problem that we must use every means in our power to prevent the products of infection being brought into contact with any member of the community.

A society has been established for this purpose the members of which intend to propagate information which will enable the laity in some measure to assist in the endeavour to control the disease. An eminent member of the profession has delivered a discourse on this subject wherein he chiefly lays stress on the danger of drinking milk and indicates the necessary means of avoiding this danger. He also recommends asses' milk as superior because less likely to be infected with tubercle. In this connexion it is interesting to note that Gideon Harvey had noticed this although he did not know the reason. Writing on the subject he says, " Asses' milk is universally preferred," and he goes on to give directions as to the diet of the ass—a matter which may or may not be of importance. In speaking of the treatment he is also very strong on the question of fresh air and change of air and also advocates change of food. "Neither it's only the change of air that proves so soveraing to Consumptives, but the change of Bread, Beer, Flesh, Company, and other circumstances do very much conduce thereunto." It is necessary to consider this question not only in the treatment, but also as a preventive, and although we are often met with the remark, " Oh! if I listen to you it is not safe to eat anything," it is nevertheless our duty to warn the public and teach them how to avoid disease. All authorities seem to be agreed upon the importance of safeguarding our food supplies, but although most elaborate precautions are taken for this purpose one of the prime sources of danger, at any rate as regards tubercle, is ignored.

Take, for instance, the inspection of bakehouses which is carried out in a fairly thorough fashion. The drains, the structure, &c., and all the appliances must be kept in a sanitary condition—i.e., in such a condition that germs will not be likely to flourish about them—but no notice is taken of the attendants, one or more of whom may be and often is suffering from phthisis, his body full of dangerous germs which are constantly fouling the atmosphere; the expectoration finds a rapid drying-ground and a temperature favourable to the life of bacilli, while the crevices in the already baked bread and other foodstuffs form a ready nidus for their reception and propagation. In these days, when hardly any bread is made in the homes, it is a question whether there is not even more danger from bread than from milk, for it is well known that phthisis is a prevalent disease amongst bakers. True, I have not got the scientific proof of my assertion and I might examine many loaves before I found tubercle bacilli. Many samples of milk might be examined with a negative result, but given the presence of tubercle bacilli in a bakehouse—and I suppose few would deny their existence there if the baker was suffering from phthisis—I do not think it is necessary to resort to scientific experiment to prove the danger. When phthisical subjects are being solemnly enjoined to carry receptacles for their sputum in order to avoid the danger of infecting the atmosphere of our towns surely there is no difficulty in realising the far greater risks in a bakehouse. Again, if it is necessary to rigidly supervise the sanitary conditions in order to ensure an atmosphere where food may be produced without fear of its being infected, surely it is approaching well nigh the ridiculous to permit an infected individual to be there present, to prepare the food, to handle it when prepared, to foul it with his exhalations and to deposit the products of his disease in and about the building. In the flour mill too phthisical workmen will often be found, and though the process of baking will perhaps sterilise the flour it is used for many other culinary purposes which may too.

Although I give the first place to bread my remarks apply to all consumable stores. If it is necessary to inspect the slaughter-house and to examine the meat, why except the butcher? Cooking should kill tubercle bacilli, but so should it destroy the eggs of the tapeworm, and yet in spite of this we annually extract many yards of this disagreeable denizen from the intestines which no doubt have been introduced in the same way as much of the tuberculous mischief finds entrance to our bodies. If ham, cheese, and butter require examination, why allow them to be retailed by a phthisical shopman? In like manner I might pass in review all articles of diet. I might even enter the sacred precincts of the domestic household and question the bodily condition of the cook and those who carry the food to the ultimate consumers. The position of safeguarding the food-supply and ignoring the condition of those who handle it seems to me a very untenable one and demands the immediate attention of those who are constituted the guardians of the public health. Will it take us as long to insist on the remedy as it has taken us to accept the fact of the infectious nature of tuberculous disease? Without expressing any disbelief in the views of Sir Richard Thorne and yourselves as expressed in your leading article of Dec. 3rd I venture to assert that the question I now raise is a point in favour of including phthisis among the dangerous infectious diseases which are compulsorily notifiable to sanitary authorities. I do not say that it proves the necessity of such an inclusion, but it does make for the necessity of investing all sanitary authorities with the power of inspecting not only the premises and the food, but also the bodies of those persons who are occupied with the food. This inspection should be no superficial formality but a rigid and thorough examination carried out at regular intervals.

In the meantime at the expense of being called an alarmist I would commend to the serious consideration of all thoughtful men the question of their food-supply. Do not be satisfied with boiling your milk; try to secure servants free from tuberculous disease and be particularly careful about your bread.

I am, Sirs, yours faithfully,

Kidderminster, Dec. 5th, 1898.   J. LIONEL STRETTON.

THE TEACHING OF ANÆSTHETICS.

To the Editors of THE LANCET.

SIRS,—Having been on the staff of a provincial hospital for nearly 20 years I have had many opportunities of observing the knowledge possessed by such recently qualified men as seek for hospital appointments. I have no hesitation in saying that the majority of them are imperfectly trained and some are lamentably ignorant in that important branch of their profession, the administration of anæsthetics. If the candidates for hospital appointments, who are generally above the average and as a rule only secure their appointments after severe competition, are deficient, the rank-and-file must be deplorably incompetent. I freely admit that I have met with notable exceptions, but I maintain that if the education was more thorough they would all be efficient, or at any rate they would not be so grossly ignorant as I have found them. For instance, I have seen men apply the facepiece of Clover's inhaler upside down. Others have commenced with the ether full on and others have admitted that they never saw the inhaler before. I have waited three-quarters of an hour while a man was endeavouring to place a patient under the influence of chloroform, and in the administration of gas I have generally had to act as instructor. Most of the men indulge in unlimited poking of their fingers into the poor patients' eyes and are generally fussy, nervous, and frightened. In a paper which I recently read before the Kidderminster Medical Society I drew attention to fright as a not unimportant element in producing a fatal termination, and I insisted upon the importance of re-assuring and obtaining the confidence of the patient at the outset. May I now add that the factor of fright on the part of the administrator is a two-fold danger, because in addition to rendering him inefficient it must react upon his patient?

I notice in your excellent article [1] that you attribute this lack of knowledge to a certain extent to the fact that the examining bodies do not demand any special training in this important subject. Your estimate is no doubt correct and the time has now arrived when the General Medical Council ought to take cognisance of the matter and insist upon a different state of affairs. To-day, almost every practitioner is called upon to give anæsthetics on frequent occasions, and his want of knowledge is not only a detriment to himself but extremely irritating to the surgeons employed and a source of much discomfort and grave danger to the patient. As a former anæsthetist at one of the largest London hospitals I have no hesitation in saying that there is ample material to give a thorough practical training to every individual student. Take the number of a year's students at St. Bartholomew's at 150, and the number of anæsthetics administered at 5000, it would certainly be a very easy matter for each student to administer 10 anæsthetics. (I should prefer 20.) My proposition is that the General Medical Council should insist that every practitioner should, before receiving his diploma, produce evidence that he has administered anæsthetics at least 20 times, including ether, gas, and chloroform, under proper supervision. There is a somewhat similar regulation with regard to confinements, so why omit the anæsthetics? There can be no question of increasing the burdens of the student. If he wishes to undertake the responsibility of administering anæsthetics surely he cannot complain if he is compelled to prove the possession of the necessary ability to do so. I hope, Sirs, the General Medical Council will give their early attention to the matter.

I am, Sirs, yours faithfully,

J. LIONEL STRETTON,
Senior Surgeon, Kidderminster Infirmary and Children's Hospital; formerly Assistant Anæsthetist, St. Bartholomew's Hospital.

Addendum 3-1: The Lancet – November 11 1900

ADDENDUM 4

KIDDERMINSTER HOSPITAL

Acknowledgements are made to
       The British Medical Journal
       for permissions to reproduce these documents.

Kidderminster Hospital Extension.

In two previous issues, April 5th, 1924 (p. 642), and March 14th, 1925 (p. 526), we referred to the scheme to increase the accommodation for children and out-patients in the Kidderminster and District General Hospital. The estimated cost of this extension was £25,000, and of this sum approximately £22,500 has now been raised. The commemoration stone of the new buildings was laid by Mrs. Stanley Baldwin on August 13th, in the unavoidable absence of the Prime Minister. The new building, which will adjoin the present block, will contain in the basement a laundry, and on the ground floor an out-patient department comprising consulting rooms, examination rooms for men and women, dressing rooms, dental rooms, a dispensary, an operating theatre, and a large waiting hall. On the first floor there will be a new ward for forty children, with an open-air balcony. Part of the old block will be converted into a nurses' dining room, an x-ray room, and servants' quarters, and over the present out-patients' department a new ward for women is to be built. The Kidderminster Hospital dates back to 1821, when a dispensary was established; in 1850 it was enlarged for the reception of in-patients. In 1870 an extensive reorganization was effected by Mr. Samuel Stretton, surgeon of the institution; his son, Mr. J. L. Stretton, now president of the hospital, is promoting the present extension scheme, and his grandson, Mr. J. W. Stretton, is surgeon to the hospital. The president is appealing for the remaining £2,500 required, and it is hoped that within the next twelve months the extensions may be opened, fully equipped, and entirely free from debt. It is believed that the cost per bed will work out at considerably less than the £400 which was the original estimate of the Voluntary Hospitals Commission.

Addendum 4-1

The British Medical Journal – August 22 1925

two medical societies and sixty-seven Panel Committees now give the Fund financial assistance.

The whole-hearted support and co-operation of the British Medical Association, together with its Branches and Divisions, and of the Medical Insurance Agency, was gratefully acknowledged. Sir Thomas Barlow said that it was very gratifying that, during the centenary celebrations of the Association, the Fund was allowed to state its case at a large conference. Dr. Lewis Glover, the treasurer, mentioned that the cost of distributing the benefits of the Fund was under 10 per cent. of the amount disbursed. The total income of the Fund during 1932 was £24,157, of which rather less than one-half was from subscriptions and donations, and rather less than one-sixth was represented by legacies. The book value of the investments stood at £155,429. Sir James Purves-Stewart proposed the adoption of the report and financial statement, and this was seconded by Mr. Bishop Harman, who mentioned the detailed personal work done by the ladies of the Ladies' Guild, which went a long way, he said, to make a success of this really lovable charity.

The re-election of Sir Thomas Barlow as president, Dr. Glover as treasurer, and Mr. Handfield Jones as honorary secretary, and of the members of the Committee of Management was voted, with thanks for their services, on motions by Dr. C. O. Hawthorne and Mr. Howard Stratford, and the president, in closing the meeting, expressed thanks to a number of individuals and bodies, including the medical journals, for publicity given to the Fund.

England and Wales

Venereal Diseases in London

The total number of new cases which were dealt with in 1932 at the hospitals utilized under the London County Council's arrangements for the diagnosis and treatment of venereal disease was 27,952, of which number 11,602 were found to be non-venereal. The new cases represent a rise of 2,000 upon the figure for 1931, when there was a decided drop, but it is pointed out that this is due almost entirely to the alteration by the Ministry of Health of the definition of a " new case," which alteration operated in the year 1931 only. The attendances numbered 983,921, as compared with 930,348 in the previous year. The new cases in 1932 included 4,941 of syphilis, 11,222 of gonorrhoea, and 187 of soft chancre. These figures, of course, are not the full measure of the extent to which venereal diseases come under treatment in London, as a not inconsiderable number of patients receive treatment by general practitioners. During 1932 no fewer than 40,626 pathological examinations were made at the hospitals at the request of and free of cost to medical practitioners for patients from all areas. The facilities afforded by the hospitals and hostels in the County of London are made use of also by the county councils of Buckingham, Essex, Hertford, Kent, Middlesex, and Surrey, and by the corporations of Croydon, East Ham, and West Ham. The L.C.C.'s participation is represented by about 79 per cent. of the whole. On the basis of the continuance of the present participation of these other authorities, provisional grants for 1933-4 amounting to £104,300 are to be made for treatment and pathological work at hospitals, and £6,600 for hostels. A sum of £2,700 will be spent on publicity and propaganda, which sum includes a grant of £2,450 to the British Social Hygiene Council. These amounts are the same as for last year.

Kidderminster General Hospital

At the annual meeting of the Kidderminster and District General Hospital Mr. J. Lionel Stretton was elected president for the tenth consecutive year, and was presented with a silver salver in recognition of his having been a member of the medical staff for fifty years. Mr. Stretton, who was born in 1860, was appointed surgeon to the hospital in 1882, and consulting surgeon in 1922, when he received a presentation from his colleagues. It was estimated by a member of the staff at the meeting that during these fifty years of service Mr. Stretton had performed about 40,000 operations, and had taken a very active part in the business side of the hospital administration. As a further tribute to his work it had been decided some months previously to raise a special testimonial fund in order to clear off the debt in connexion with the new nurses' home and other extensions, and a sum of more than £1,750 has already been subscribed. The mayor remarked that the hospital was itself a monument to its president, whose untiring optimism and zeal had prevailed against the many depressing influences of recent years. The annual report showed a slight financial deficit, which was less than that in previous years ; no further administrative economies seemed to be practicable, for the hospital was working at its extreme capacity, and 108 out of its 124 beds were occupied on the average each day. The president, in his speech, concluded that it had become necessary to increase the weekly contributions from twopence to threepence. He did not doubt that the additional support would be forthcoming, although the present economic difficulties were being severely felt in the town. During the previous year these weekly contributors had raised £7,000, and this figure would be increased by about £3,000 if the extra penny rate was generally accepted. Mr. Stretton commented also on the difficulties in obtaining payment for patients admitted to hospital in consequence of motor car accidents. It was often impossible to secure any sums from the insurance societies concerned, owing to the present state of the law relating to such liabilities. In order to meet the various financial requirements the cost of maintenance at the hospital had been reduced to about two guineas a week, which was far below that of some other comparable institutions. The advance of science had necessitated more expenditure on equipment, and the hospital had kept pace with others in this respect also. Mr. Stretton concluded with a warm expression of appreciation of the work of other members of the hospital team, and in this connexion it may be mentioned that he has been three times chairman of the Worcestershire Division of the British Medical Association.

Public Health Congress at Eastbourne

The annual congress of the Royal Institute of Public Health will be held this year at Eastbourne from Tuesday, May 30th, to Sunday, June 4th. There will be five Sections—namely : State medicine and industrial hygiene ; women and children and the public health ; tuberculosis ; pathology, bacteriology, biochemistry, and veterinary medicine ; and hydrology and climatology. Sir Allan Powell, president of the first-named Section, will deliver an address on changes and prospects in the public health field ; this will be followed by a discussion on the pure milk problem. Sir Josiah Stamp will speak on the economic test of the limits of public health expenditure ; and other topics to be considered are the housing problem, industrial welfare under existing conditions, and the principles and practice of health education. Dame Louise McIlroy, president of the second Section, will give a lecture on a maternity service within the reach of patients of moderate means. Other subjects to be dealt with in this Section are the role of the midwife in a national maternity service (opened by Sir Ewen Maclean), biology as a basis for teaching sex hygiene to children, and the study and care of exceptional children. Sir P. Varrier-Jones, president of the Section of Tuberculosis, will deliver an address on the question why this disease still remains a

Addendum 4-2: The British Medical Journal – April 1 1933

ADDENDUM 5

MISCELLANEOUS

5-1   Ambulance conveyances in London
The British Medical Journal – July 30 1881

5-2   The difficulty in obtaining information from the General Medical Council
The Lancet – October 24 1896

5-3   School punishments
The Lancet – November 30 1901

5-4   Feeding babies in crèches
The British Medical Journal – June 23 1906

5-5   Experiments on live animals
The British Medical Journal – March 28 1908

5-6   Motor cars: spare parts
The British Medical Journal – November 19 1921

5-7   Motor cars: spare parts
The British Medical Journal – November 26 1921

Acknowledgements are made to
The British Medical Journal and The Lancet
for permissions to reproduce these documents.

AMBULANCE CONVEYANCES IN LONDON.

SIR,—I am glad to note your article upon Dr. B. Howard's letter, asserting the great need for ambulance conveyances for the sick and wounded in London.

Two months ago, I was summoned to town to find a medical student (my son) in great danger, with diphtheritic throat; and, feeling his life could only be saved by an immediate removal from his lodgings to hospital care, I cast about for a proper conveyance. Various messengers were sent to different owners of the same; at last, one was found willing to undertake the removal, a distance under a mile. He would not show his vehicle, or promise it, before a deposit of ten shillings was made. On its arrival, I was in dismay; the landlady and the whole square deeply shocked at the sight of the conveyance. I can only describe it as a cross between a hearse and dirty linen cart, painted black, and with funereal side glass; a black horse, with dismal harness, and a driver of the most woeful aspect, also in deep black. It was surely enough to put the finish to any sensitive patient, dangerously ill, as my son then was. Surely, in these days, the metropolis will not long delay this much needed proper ambulance provision.—I am, faithfully yours,

SAMUEL STRETTON, M.R.C.S.Eng.

Kidderminster, July, 1881.

Addendum 5-1

The British Medical Journal – July 30 1881

THE DIFFICULTY OF OBTAINING INFORMATION FROM THE GENERAL MEDICAL COUNCIL.

To the Editors of THE LANCET.

SIRS,—A few days ago I applied to the Registrar of the General Medical Council to ascertain if a certain gentleman was qualified because I could not find his name in the Register, and I thought it possible it had been added since its publication. I was anxious to know whether it would be correct to associate myself with him in consultation or otherwise, for although it is generally held that we are blameless for meeting a man who professes to be qualified it has always seemed to me to be a duty to the profession and the public to ascertain the genuineness of such qualifications. The reply I received was an "inquiry form," and I could not quite make out why I should be put to the unnecessary trouble of re-writing my queries on a form until I perceived the following footnote :—

"The Registrar may supply information in regard to registration provided only that he should deem it consistent with his duty to do so. In case the Registrar should think fit to supply the required information he will forward it on receiving from an applicant the above form, duly filled up, together with the prescribed inquiry fee of 2s. 6d. The information thus furnished may be used as evidence, in accordance with the subjoined section of the Medical Act (1886)."

To answer me would not have involved so much trouble as sending the form. It appears, then, that this wealthy body, which expends vast sums of money on its meetings, whose most important duty is to regulate the behaviour of the profession, refuses to answer a question which will assist in improving that behaviour unless it is applied for a second time on a form and accompanied by half-a-crown. I maintain that when the General Medical Council thus throws obstacles in the way of our obtaining information it thwarts the detection of offenders. It is their duty to afford every facility to anyone who will take the trouble to ask for information and not to discourage the few who are willing to write for guidance ; in any case the paltry fee of half-a-crown should not prevent them answering a question which may assist in the prevention of the abuses they profess to abhor.

Now that the election is in the air perhaps some of the would-be representatives will take this matter up.

I am, Sirs, yours faithfully,

Kidderminster, Oct. 20th, 1896.   J. LIONEL STRETTON.

Addendum 5-2: The Lancet – October 24 1986

SCHOOL PUNISHMENTS.

To the Editors of THE LANCET.

SIRS,—I have been very interested in the correspondence which has lately appeared in THE LANCET with reference to the above subject. While there is much to commend many of the views which have been put forward I do not think a sufficient case has been made out for the adoption of a special system or the abolition of any of the methods which have been discussed. At the present day we have become such victims to fashion that it permeates into our lives and affects our actions more than we care to admit. Religion itself is not free from its effects. In the legitimate branch of our own profession it exerts a baneful influence and on the illegitimate side the harm it does is appalling. Yesterday it was Count Mattei, to-day it is the violet leaves, and to-morrow who knows what it will be? We must be careful in considering the punishment of our young people not to allow ourselves to be swayed by such an influence.

In choosing methods of punishment I cannot help thinking that it would be a wise plan to endeavour as far as possible (if I may use a well-known phrase) "to make the punishment fit the crime." For instance, while, on the one hand, I should not approve of a form of punishment which kept a lad indoors and so deprived him of the necessary fresh air and physical exercise, on the other hand it appears to me that if a boy fails to learn his lesson the natural punishment is to keep him in after school hours while he does learn it. It is probable that instead of devoting the time he should have devoted to the preparation of his lesson he was playing about, perhaps out-of-doors, so that in the end you will not deprive him of his necessary exercise. Of course, in such a system it is essential that the master should sufficiently gauge the capacity of his pupil so that he may not be set a task beyond his ability. Corporal punishment should be reserved for really serious sins, such as untruthfulness, theft, immoral practices, &c., and should be administered with some degree of comparison to the offence. No one, I think, can defend the system of ear-boxing, pinching, pin-pricking, or roasting, and the old custom of slashing boys on the hands is equally to be condemned. It is far better for their bodies and more humiliating to their minds if the punishment is inflicted upon that portion of their body which nature appears to have specially designed for that purpose. The object of this punishment is to produce pain without damaging the soft parts, consequently it should never be performed with a fine cane, which is liable to cut the skin, nor should it be applied to the skin without any covering or in too rough or too extensive a manner. If the recipient is made to kneel down and a good thick cane be used half a dozen smart stripes could rarely do harm. Boys have a great idea of justice, and providing that this is exercised they will generally accept their punishment in a proper spirit and profit by it, but I should like in conclusion to put in a plea for the personal factor. Every boy is a study in himself, and if a master observes his pupils as he ought he will soon ascertain that a form of punishment which is most suitable to one boy is totally unsuited to another. While I should like to feel that all could be dispensed with I am sure that it would be most undesirable to fix upon any one method, and the wise master is he who makes use of them all in the cases to which they are applicable.

I am, Sirs, yours faithfully,

J. LIONEL STRETTON,

Senior Surgeon to the Kidderminster Infirmary and Children's Hospital.

Nov. 26th, 1901.

Addendum 5-3: The Lancet – November 30 1901

FEEDING BABIES IN CRÈCHES.

Sir,—Your article on the above reminds me of a letter I received a short time ago from a relative of mine who resides in Alexandria. The following extract from it will, I think, be an interesting contribution to the subject :

A few days ago I went to the Maternity Home in Alexandria. They have lately started a crèche there for deserted babies and those of utterly destitute mothers. Everthing was spotlessly clean. Six babies, all under 3 months, lay in six little white bassinettes. It was just feeding time. I saw a strange sight. A clean, plump goat was laid on its side on a bed between clean sheets, and the babies went to it in turn and drank away happily. The babies are plump and rosy, need no medicine, rarely cry; just drink and sleep. Next time a different goat would be brought. The matron said it was a much safer system and much less trouble than bottles. Some of the babies were so tiny that they were kept in incubators, taken out only when put to the goat.

—I am, etc.,   J. Lionel Stretton,

June 18th.   Senior Surgeon. Kidderminster Infirmary and
                              Children's Hospital.

Addendum 5-4

The British Medical Journal – June 23 1906

EXPERIMENTS ON LIVE ANIMALS.

SIR,—In an account of the fire at Hamstead Colliery published in the *Birmingham Gazette and Express* for Friday, March 6th, it is reported:

A continuous stream of water was poured into the main shaft, and the effect of this was shown when, at 8 o'clock yesterday morning, a linnet was let down in a cage into that shaft and allowed to remain for five or ten minutes. On being brought to the surface it was alive, and this gave some hope that the worst might be over and that the poor fellows who had been cut off from communication with the outer world might still be rescued.

In the issue of the same paper for the previous day I believe it was stated that a rat was let down in a similar way to ascertain if it could live in the atmosphere.

There is no evidence that those who performed these experiments possessed any licence, and it appears from the report that no anaesthetic was administered.

It is not definitely stated by whom the experiments were performed, but it seems probable that several prominent men witnessed it, and it is possible that one of these may have been His Majesty's Inspector of Mines, who is stated to be in attendance.

These poor animals were sent down the shaft with the full knowledge that they might have to suffer the tortures of suffocation, or perhaps be roasted alive, without any chance of protest or escape. For what reason? In order to save the life, or, more correctly, to save discomfort to a human being. The latter would be able to signal to the pit's mouth to be brought up if danger occurred, while the poor dumb creature could not.

And yet there is no word of protest, no question to the Home Secretary, and no motion for the adjournment of the House of Commons to discuss the question! One would have expected a torrent of protest from a Society which is so conspicuous in its condemnation of scientific research. One could even have imagined the arrival of a trainload of their members ready to volunteer their service rather than allow such cruelty.

It certainly appears strange that a medical man is not allowed to perform an experiment, even under an anaesthetic, without a licence, and then is condemned by the above mentioned Society. The fact that his experiment may save much suffering and perhaps many lives is no justification. And yet, in order to save possible discomfort to one person, animals can be subjected to the possibility of being roasted alive without protest.— I am, etc.,

J. LIONEL STRETTON,
Senior Surgeon, Kidderminster Infirmary and
Children's Hospital.
Kidderminster, March 8th.

Addendum 5-5: The British Medical Journal – March 28 1908

MOTOR CARS: SPARE PARTS.

SIR,—There is one very important point with regard to the choice of a motor car which your expert has not touched upon.

It is the supply of spare parts. Many of your readers may not be aware that some of the British motor firms refuse to send these parts until they have been paid for. I remember on one occasion writing for a part which was valued at about 30s. I explained in my letter how necessary it was, as I required the use of the car for my professional work, and I could not drive it until the part arrived. I asked for it to be sent by the first train next morning and said my man would meet it. They did not send it. They did not even trouble to telegraph to me. They wrote a letter stating that the price of the part was 30s., and that on receipt of the amount it should be dispatched. This involved a delay of three days with its attendant worry and expense.

Nothing would induce me to purchase another car from this firm, and I would strongly advise any member of the profession, before placing an order for a car, to insist on a guarantee that spare parts shall be dispatched immediately on receipt of request.—I am, etc.,

J. LIONEL STRETTON,
Consulting Surgeon, Kidderminster Infirmary and Children's Hospital.

November 8th.

Addendum 5-6: The British Medical Journal – November 19 1921

MOTOR CARS: SPARE PARTS.

SIR,—Dr. Lionel Stretton has written a much-needed warning on this subject (p. 868), but I go further and warn my brother medicos against dealing with firms that cannot supply spare parts at all.

Only last week, on applying for spares to the London agent for an excellent French car, I was disgusted to receive a wire, "Regret cannot supply parts."

I have written to them and pointed out that, however excellent a car is, it is useless unless one can replace parts, and that in future I shall be unable to recommend their cars.

The local garage manager informs me he has the same difficulty with all makes except the Americans. Is it anything to be wondered at that our makers are given the "go-by"?—I am, etc.,

GEORGE P. BLETCHLY, M.B.Lond.

Nailsworth, Gloucestershire, Nov. 19th.

Addendum 5-7: The British Medical Journal – November 26 1921

ADDENDUM 6

THE AMBULANCE LECTURES

6-1   A course of Ambulance Lectures, delivered in Kidderminster
by John Lionel Stretton, L.R.C.P., Lond.: M.R.C.S. and L.S.A. Eng
1889

Title page and PrefaceAddendum 6-

A COURSE OF

AMBULANCE

LECTURES

Delivered in Kidderminster,

BY

J. LIONEL STRETTON,

L.R.C.P., LOND.; M.R.C.S. AND L.S.A. ENG.

Hon. Surgeon Kidderminster Infirmary and Children's Hospital;
Surgeon Kidderminster Maternity Charity;
Hon. Physician Midland Counties Home for Chronic and
Incurable Diseases;
Hon. Surgeon Station Ambulance Corps, Kidderminster;
Examiner and Honorary Life Member St. John Ambulance
Association;
Member Medical Council St. John's House, Worcester;
Member Abernethian Society;
Formerly Assistant Chloroformist St. Bartholomew's Hospital,
London.

KIDDERMINSTER :
PRINTED BY W. HEPWORTH, BULL RING.
1889.

1

PREFACE.

ALTHOUGH many books on Ambulance Work are already published, I have ventured to thus arrange the notes of my Lectures, chiefly that those who have hitherto studied with me, and those who will in the future do so, may be able to follow me the more easily. With the growing importance of Ambulance Work, I feel sure that there is room for yet other useful books on the subject, and I trust that this may be counted amongst that number. It may also serve as a guide to those called upon, for the first time, to 'deliver such a Course of Lectures. I have selected only two illustrations which I consider essential for an understanding of my remarks; my reason being partly because I am convinced that nothing but practice will ensure a thorough knowledge of the various appliances and movements, and partly because I am anxious to publish these Lectures in a cheap form. I lay claim to little originality, the subject matter of the book having of necessity been, in a large measure, derived from earlier works.

ADDENDUM 7

APPRECIATIONS & OBITUARY

Acknowledgements are made to
   The Kidderminster Shuttle, The British Medical Journal
   and Express Newspapers
   for permissions to reproduce these documents.

"SHUTTLE" PORTRAIT
GALLERY NO. 2

MR. JOHN LIONEL STRETTON, J.P.

No man in Kidderminster and district has done more for his fellow members of the community in the relief of sickness and suffering than Mr. John Lionel Stretton, J.P., who for over 50 years was on the staff as an honorary surgeon at Kidderminster General Hospital, and who has performed more than 40,000 operations. Although now aged 81, Mr. Stretton is as robust and vigorous as ever, both in mind and body.

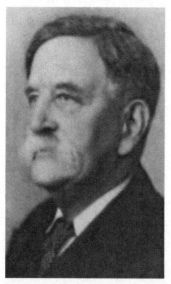

When the "Shuttle" representative called upon him to wish him a Happy New Year and to ask him the favour of an interview for the paper he found the. celebrated surgeon in his consulting room, on the walls of which were hung portraits of distinguished surgeons, many of whom Mr Stretton had known personally during his long career in the medical profession. Perhaps the most notable is a portrait of Lord Lister, the British surgeon and scientist, whose constant advocacy of antiseptics marked one of the greatest advances in surgery. Another picture was of Dr. John Abernethy, the famous surgeon who first enunciated the principle that local diseases were symptomatic.

Mr. Stretton is the third generation of surgeons in his family and his son, Mr. John W. Stretton represents the fourth generation.

Mr. J. L. Stretton was born at Elderfield House, Kidderminster, on September 20th, 1860. His father Mr. Samuel Stretton, after being a surgeon in the Crimean War - where he met Florence Nightingale - came to Kidderminster in 1856.

CAREER AT BARTS

The subject of our sketch was educated at King Charles I Grammar School of which he is now a governor, and after being apprenticed to the late Dr. Cecil Webster, of Bewdley, he went to St. Bartholomew's Hospital London, where he met students who became famous in later life and many who were already famous including the great Lord Lister of King's College Hospital and Dr W G Grace, the cricketer, who trained with him at St. Bartholomew's. When at St. Bartholomew's Hospital Mr. Stretton was appointed assistant anaesthetist and resident gynaecologist and house surgeon, positions he relinquished to join his father. In the competitive examinations the then young Mr Stretton was first in physiology second in anatomy and second in surgical scholarship. He also won a prize dressership. In 1882 Mr Stretton joined his father in partnership in Kidderminster and in 1904 Mr S. Stretton, after having practised for 56 years, retired. Thus Mr Stretton's father, his grandfather and his son have all been St. Bartholomew's Hospital men, so there have been four generations of the family there. Another unique family event is that Mr Stretton's grandfather, his father and himself have all celebrated their golden weddings and Mr. Stretton was present at all three events. His grandfather Mr William Weston Stretton, J.P. of Leicester, celebrated his golden wedding in 1876, his father, Mr Samuel Stretton, J.P., of Kidderminster celebrated his golden wedding on April 28th 1907 and Mr Stretton celebrated his golden wedding on April 21st 1934.

Mr. Stretton married Miss Lucy Emma Houghton younger daughter of the late Mr. J Freeth Houghton, of Park Hill, Moseley and the wedding took place at St Anne's Church Moseley. Birmingham on April 21st 1884. His maternal grandfather was the late Mr William Birch, a surgeon of Barton-under-Needwood, near Burton-on-Trent. Mr. Stretton was appointed an honorary surgeon to Kidderminster Hospital in December 1882, on the retirement of his father, and for about 56 years carried out operations there until his retirement in 1938. In 1933, on the completion of 50 years at the hospital, Mr Stretton was presented with a beautiful Chippendale salver engraved as follows: "Presented to J. Lionel Stretton Esq., J.P., by the friends and supporters of Kidderminster and District General Hospital on the occasion of his completing 50 years as a member of the honorary medical staff in recognition of the long, devoted and valuable services rendered to the people of the town and district, 1882-1932." At the same time Mr. Stretton was given a cheque for £1,700 which was handed over to the hospital. When this presentation was made Mr Stretton said he felt he owed a deep debt of gratitude to his parents. His father was the mainspring in bringing about the present hospital buildings and his mother had been a constant help-meet to his father in that work.

HOSPITAL IMPROVEMENTS

During his career at Kidderminster Hospital Mr. Stretton brought about many improvements and developments among which was the establishment of a children's ward, the money for which was given by his uncle the late Sir Thomas Lea. Bart., the erection of the Godson Memorial Chapel, by public subscription and the installation of the X-ray apparatus which was opened by Sir Malcolm Morris, the famous skin specialist from London and a pioneer in X-ray work. The subscriptions for the latter were collected by Lady Lea, wife of Sir Thomas Sydney Lea, Bart. who is a cousin of Mr. Stretton. After this was the building of an Isolation Ward since converted into a pathological department from funds raised by public subscription. Then there was the Victoria Memorial which consisted of building of an operating theatre, under what is the William Adams ward, presented by the late Mrs William in memory of her husband, who was the grandfather of Mr. Raleigh R. Adam the present President of the hospital. Subsequently the trend of progress led to the building of two isolation wards given by an anonymous friend of Mr. Stretton, and then the King Edward Memorial which consisted of the purchase of Needwood House and its conversion into a nursing home. The funds for this were collected by Mr. J. Johnson, a former president of the hospital. Beginning with the gift of £5.000 from Mr. Stanley Baldwin an extension scheme was put into operation and through the organising genius of Mr. Stretton, the public subscriptions reached £35,000 which paid for an out-patients' department and two children's wards and a model laundry which were opened by the present King when he was Duke of York on July 21st. 1926. The next thing was an increase to the nurses home which Mr. Thomas Griffin, J.P. gave in memory of his wife at a cost of £5,000. Mr. Stretton gave the "Sunnyside" Nursing Home and a field contiguous to the hospital and has raised a fund of £7,000 which he hopes will be used to carry out further extensions when the present war is over.

HONOURS FROM HIS PROFESSION

In December 1933, Mr. Stretton was honoured by members of his profession from all parts of Worcestershire at a complimentary dinner given at Kidderminster to celebrate his 21st year as chairman of the County of Worcester Local Medical and Panel Committee. Representatives of the Ministry of Health and of Worcestershire Health Insurance Committee were present. At that dinner Mr Stretton was presented with a silver dessert service by the members of that committee

In December 1932, Mr. Stretton's colleagues on the honorary medical staff presented him with a silver dessert dish on completion of 50 years' active service as surgeon at the hospital. The Matron and nurses gave him a silver cigar box.

Among many other gifts are some from patients whose lives have been saved through Mr. Stretton operating upon them. After the last war the members of Kidderminster Medical Society gave Mr. Stretton a gold cigarette case. He was the first medical referee to be appointed at Kidderminster under the Workmen's Compensation Act and in order that he would be able to deal with the cases properly Mr. Stretton descended the Highley coal pit and walked to the face, a distance of a mile and a half. Mr Stretton is a former chairman of Worcestershire Division of the British Medical Association and has also been chairman of the Worcestershire and Herefordshire branch of that Association. For 30 years he has been chairman of the Local Medical Society and for over 40 years chairman of the local Public Medical Club.

On January 29th, 1921, a public banquet was given in Mr. Stretton's honour by the Worcestershire Division of the British Medical Association when he was presented with a silver salver in recognition of his valuable services and of the esteem in which he is held. In addition to being honorary consulting surgeon Mr. Stretton was President of Kidderminster Hospital from 1924 to 1938 when he resigned from that position. A portrait of Mr. Stretton was hung in the Board Room of the hospital, subscribed for by his colleagues on the staff. Mr. Stretton comes of a long lived family, for his grandfather lived to be 92 and his father 89 years of age.

A GREAT DISCOVERY

One of Mr. Stretton's proudest achievements was that after long experiments and research at Kidderminster Hospital he discovered the method of the sterilisation of the skin by the use of tincture of iodine B.P. which was published in the "British Medical Journal," the official organ of the British Medical Association, in August, 1909. This method of skin sterilisation has been adopted throughout the world.

Mr. Stretton entered the Town Council in 1888 and was the first member for Rowland Hill Ward after the town was divided. He served for three years and in order to become thoroughly acquainted with his duties Mr. Stretton walked through the main sewer of Kidderminster from the premises of Carpet Trades Ltd., to the Town Hall. In walking through Mr. Stretton found that the brickwork had given way in several places leaving large cavities which resembled cesspools. He suggested that these should be filled up with concrete so that the sewage could pass freely but no notice was taken of his suggestion though the work has been done since. Mr Stretton also descended the upper well on the Stouport Road in a loop of rope 150 feet long and found everything satisfactory. While a member of the Town Council Mr Stretton was horrified to find three or four families huddled together sleeping in lodging houses in the same room. He advocated the erection of model lodging houses and, when this was not adopted, purchased the Hill House, Orchard Street, which he had converted into a model lodging house which has now been run for over 30 years by his ex-chauffeur, Mr. H. Teale.

DROVE IN A BROUGHAM

Mr. Stretton up to two years ago always wore the traditional top silk hat of the medical profession and for many years visited his patients, who lived in all parts of the county, by driving in a Brougham or Victoria. He kept as many as seven horses at one time and in one year so extensive was his practice that he drove over 10,000 miles. He was the first driver of a motor-car in Kidderminster but had so much trouble with it that he had to get rid of it and return to his horses. In the height of his career patients came to Mr. Stretton from London, Birmingham, U.S.A., Canada, Australia, New Zealand, and South Africa. Mr. Stretton has also taken a very active part in ambulance work and the training of nurses. In 1890 he was appointed an honorary associate of the Order of St. John of Jerusalem. He has been a justice of the peace since 1922.

When Professor Koch discovered tuberculin, Mr. Stretton visited Berlin and saw him, together with Professor Virchow and several other eminent German specialists.

During the Great War Mr. Stretton had wounded soldiers continuously under his care in the hospital.

"I have not had a holiday for 30 years." said Mr Stretton, "and an exaggerated value is placed on holidays. Many people go away for a holiday to make themselves ill because they indulge in all manner of excesses. Holidays have an advantage from an educational point of view rather than a health point of view. There are three advantages in a holiday: (1) anticipation, (2) the realisation, and (3) the most important of all, contemplation, because nothing can deprive one of the beautiful scenery which one enjoys on a holiday." Mr Stretton added that the value of exercise was often overestimated. The late Sir William Jenner, physician to Queen Victoria, asked his opinion of the craze for exercise, said: "I only walk from my front door to my Brougham and I would not walk that far if I could get someone to carry me." Jenner lived to be 89 years old.

288

SPORTING PROCLIVITIES

In sport Mr. Stretton was fond of cricket and football and in the latter game played quarter back for Kidderminster Rugby Club in 1876 and 1877. He also used to ride an old "boneshaker" to Worcester, and after that a "penny-farthing" machine on which he once rode to Manchester. For seven years Mr. Stretton was chairman of the Old Carolians. He was also chairman of the Kidderminster Horse Parade and show and afterwards of the Cycle Parade, which later was converted into the Carnival. For over 40 years Mr. Stretton was honorary secretary of the Church Street and Brecknell Charity. He was a frequent attender at the Burns dinner at Stourport as a guest of his friend, Dr. Brocket. During the last war Mr. Stretton was chairman of the local Medical War Committee for the County of Worcester and is chairman of the present one.

In 1883 there was an epidemic of smallpox in the town, with over 100 cases, and Bromsgrove Street was boarded up to prevent people going down it. Two wooden hospitals were erected in the grounds of the workhouse and Mr. Stretton had charge of these. About a year later there was an epidemic of enteric fever, when Mr. Stretton had 500 sufferers under his care.

Asked what his opinion was about the future of hospitals. Mr. Stretton said: "I am afraid the profession and the hospitals will be taken over by the State, but I do not think it will be for the benefit of the public because it will take away the human side of medicine and surgery and the patients will not receive the same personal interest in their cases." Mr. Stretton has two sons, Mr. Samuel Stretton who is married to the matron of the Kidderminster hospital and Mr. John W. Stretton, a surgeon and hon. senior surgeon at the hospital. His daughter and eldest child is Mrs. Davis, wife of Canon Claude Davis, of Abington, Northants. His son, Mr John W. Stretton, has three sons and his daughter, Mrs. Davis, has three daughters.

On the occasion of the celebration of his golden wedding, Mr. Stretton paid the following tribute to his wife: "Further-more I have the comfort of a good wife who has helped me in my duties for the hospital and I feel it is, only right that on this occasion I should refer to that."

Addendum 7.3: Kidderminster Shuttle – January 10 1942

JOHN LIONEL STRETTON, M.R.C.S., J.P.

We regret to announce the death at the age of 82 on Feb. 14 after a few days' illness of Dr. J. L. Stretton, honorary consulting surgeon to the Kidderminster and District General Hospital. Born at Kidderminster in 1860, John Lionel Stretton received his medical education at St. Bartholomew's Hospital, and qualified M.R.C.S. in 1881. In the following year he took the L.R.C.P. and the L.S.A. He was appointed assistant anaesthetist at St. Bartholomew's and was to have been resident gynaecologist and house-surgeon, but he returned home to join his father's practice. In 1882 he succeeded his father as an honorary surgeon to the Kidderminster Hospital and was an active member of the staff for 56 years. When he resigned at the end of 1938 he accepted the position of honorary consulting surgeon. He was president of the hospital from 1924 to 1937. His professional ability and administrative skill were of incalculable value to the hospital, and his work for it was a dominating factor in his life. His method of sterilizing the skin with iodine was described in the *Journal* in 1909 and 1910 and afterwards generally adopted. The most remarkable of his pathological specimens were exhibited before the war in the Wellcome Museum in London, where they are now in safe keeping. In 1936 Mr. Stretton gave his private nursing-home, with its equipment, to the hospital, to be used for paying patients.

He was a Justice of the Peace, and other offices he held included that of chairman of the Worcestershire Division of the B.M.A. in 1911, 1912, 1916, and 1920, and president of the Worcestershire and Herefordshire Branch (1914) ; chairman of the Local Medical Committee for the County of Worcester (1914-18) ; chairman of the Local Medical War Committee for the Worcester and Bromsgrove area (1939-42) ; chairman of the County of Worcester Local Medical and Panel Committee (1912-42) ; and president of the Kidderminster Medical Society. A man of sound judgment and strong views, he was inflexible in upholding what he considered right. His guiding principles were self-sacrificing devotion and unswerving loyalty to his ideals, his profession, and his friends. He leaves a widow, two sons, and a daughter ; the younger son, John W. Stretton, F.R.C.S., is senior honorary surgeon to the Kidderminster Hospital, and thus represents the third generation of his family on the staff.

Addendum 7-2: The British Medical Journal — March 13 1943

| **ALAN TOMKINS'** Inquiring Mind discovers

The Man Who Made the World say *'Oh!'*

MILLIONS of Britons during the past 30 years have cried "*Oh!*"—all because of a man who died, almost unnoticed, last Sunday.

With regret I recall the howls of pain he made me utter, and the flow of really very, very bad language.

Brief obituary notices said that John Lionel Stretton, who died at Kidderminster, aged 82, discovered the method of sterilisation of the skin by the use of tincture of iodine.

Until recently iodine was used in every home for cuts and scratches, and in the last war an ampoule was in every soldier's field dressing.

So I cornered one of the senior of my numerous medical friends and said: "Was not this a tremendous contribution to medicine? Ought not Mr. Stretton to be almost as well known as Lister?"

"Undoubtedly," he said. "When I started, in 1901, preparing a patient for, say, an abdominal operation meant a great deal of fuss and bother and delay.

"A student would wash a patient, shave him, wash him again with ether soap, sponge him down with biniodide of mercury, and apply a compress of carbolic.

"This would take half a day.

"Then on the morning of the operation a nurse would do the whole job again.

"Stretton's method made a dramatic change. All this fuss and

dragging the patient about was superseded by painting the surrounding skin with tincture of iodine, which took a few seconds.

"Many old surgeons suspected the new method. I remember a colleague of mine who assisted at an old-method operation saying. 'The old boy made me wash my hands in 10 poisons and then wear rubber gloves.'

"The iodine caused irritation in some skins. One school began to use only the spirit in which the iodine was dissolved, but this led to the complaint that, as there was no stain, the surgeon could not be sure that the affected part had been treated.

"Iodine has been superseded in surgery by picric acid, flavine, and other antiseptics, but it has been of immense benefit to surgery."

★

I WENT to the War Office and asked if they still used iodine ampoules.

"No," they said very politely. "We gave that up at the end of the last war. For a time we issued euflavine with the field dressings. Now our people prefer a dressing which has been specially treated and sealed, so that it may be applied at once to the wound."

So I went to the British Medical Association's forbidding palace, which houses kind hearts, and asked for copies of the *British Medical Journal* for the exciting time when Mr. Stretton was revolutionising hospital routine.

Browsing through the files of 1909 and 1910, I found that lots of

patients got eczema from "over-preparation" for operations, and that Dr. A. Grossich, of Fiume, and Professor von Eiselberg, of Vienna, were trying iodine coincidentally with Mr. Stretton.

On August 14, 1909, Mr. Stretton wrote of causes of suppuration for which surgeons were unable to account. "Of all our preparations," he said, "the one least under control is sterilisation of the skin."

Apparently foreign experiments had been made with 10 per cent solution of iodine. "I could not bring myself to paint such a strong solution," he recalls, and gives the history of his first cases with a solution one quarter that strength.

★

IN the first two months he tried 50 minor cases, and in the second two months 84. Then he tried iodine for 57 operations, of which six were satisfactory and the rest "perfect."

He made these claims for his method:

The surgeon was certain that the method had been completed.

It was quick and easily applied

It saved suffering and disagreeable preparation,

It obviated shaving (except where a shaven surface would help the actual operation).

It had great value in emergency.

When the method was widely adopted, one surgeon wrote in mournfully and said that he had used it first but, alas, had written nothing about it

In 1910 Mr Stretton wrote that the 10 per cent solution used by Grossich "caused excessive lacrymation in the surgeon and his assistants," a very sad picture, you will agree.

A few diehards attacked the system because of the irritation and swelling created in a small percentage of patients, but the truth was that these irritations caused by iodine were slight against the irritation caused by the old, tedious methods.

And that, Dear Reader, was Mr. Stretton, without whom a good many of us running around now would have been dead many years ago.

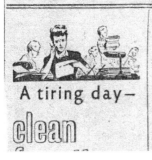

A tiring day—

clean

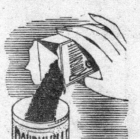

Addendum 7-3: Sunday Dispatch – 21 February 1943

ADDENDUM 8

PUBLICATION REJECTION

8-1   William Heinemann letter

WILLIAM HEINEMANN
(MEDICAL BOOKS)
LTD.
J. • A. ELLIOT, M.A.
Chairman and Managing Director
Directors
J. JOHNSTON ABRAHAM
C. S. EVANS
A. S. FRERE-REEVES M.A (CANTAB)
H. I. HALL
B. F. OLIVER
Secretary
W. de LANGLOIS IRISE
Telegraphic Address:
"SUNLOCKS LONDON"
Telephone:
MUSEUM (0944 (4 Lines)

MEDICAL, SURGICAL, DENTAL & SCIENTIFIC PUBLISHERS.

99 GREAT RUSSELL STREET,
LONDON, W.C.1.

April 25th, 1940.

Miss Susan Smith,
Roden House,
19 Roden Avenue,
KIDDERMINSTER.

Dear Madam,

We have now had a report from our reader on
Mr. Lionel Stretton's book FIFTY-SIX YEARS A SURGEON.
His opinion is that while it is a very interesting
production and has much historical value, it would be
more interesting fifty years hence than now. He cannot
recommend us to publish it as he does not think that
at the present time it would have much commercial value.
I am, therefore, returning the MS. under separate cover,
and if Mr. Stretton would like to consider the publication
of the book at his own expense we shall be very glad to
give you an estimate for the same and pay 15% commission
on any sales.

Yours faithfully,

WILLIAM HEINEMANN (MEDICAL BOOKS) LTD.

Hugh Elliot
MANAGING DIRECTOR.

Lightning Source UK Ltd.
Milton Keynes UK
UKOW050648060613

211784UK00008B/171/P